Dating Someone with a Personality Disorder

The Complete Guide to All 10 Disorders and Building Healthy Relationships

Crystal Kita Logan

Table of Contents

Chapter 1: You're Not Alone

The phone rings at 2 AM again. Your heart pounds as you wonder what crisis waits on the other end. Maybe it's another accusation, another tearful breakdown, or another threat to leave. You answer because you love them, but each call chips away at something inside you. Sound familiar? You're holding this book because something in your relationship feels different from what others describe—more intense, more confusing, more exhausting than typical relationship problems.

The Hidden Epidemic

10-15% of People Have Personality Disorders

The numbers tell a story that most people never hear. According to the Merck Manual and multiple psychiatric studies, personality disorders affect between 10-15% of the adult population. That means roughly 1 in 8 people you encounter lives with patterns of thinking and behaving that significantly impact their relationships. Yet somehow, this information stays locked away in medical journals and clinical settings, leaving partners like you to navigate these challenges alone.

Consider what this means practically. In a room of 100 people, 10-15 of them have personality disorders. In your neighborhood, workplace, or social circle, these conditions exist more commonly than diabetes, which affects about 11% of adults. But while diabetes has awareness campaigns, support groups, and clear treatment protocols, personality disorders remain shrouded in secrecy and shame.

The Merck Manual identifies ten distinct personality disorders, each creating unique challenges for both the person with the condition and their loved ones. These aren't character flaws or choices—

1

they're deeply ingrained patterns that typically develop during childhood and adolescence. Understanding this distinction changes everything about how you approach your relationship.

Case Example 1 Maria's Wake-Up Call Maria dated Kevin for three years before she realized something fundamental was different about their relationship dynamic. Kevin would alternate between intense devotion and cold withdrawal, creating a cycle that left Maria constantly anxious and confused. When she mentioned this to friends, they offered typical relationship advice: "Just communicate better" or "He must be stressed at work." But their suggestions never addressed the underlying pattern.

After a particularly intense episode where Kevin accused Maria of cheating (despite having no evidence), she started researching and discovered information about borderline personality disorder. The descriptions matched Kevin's behavior patterns perfectly—the fear of abandonment, the intense relationships, the emotional instability. For the first time, Maria had a framework to understand what was happening. She wasn't crazy, oversensitive, or inadequate as a partner. She was dealing with a complex mental health condition that required specific strategies and understanding.

Your Story Matters

Validating Partner Experiences Across All Disorders

Every relationship touched by a personality disorder creates its own unique story of confusion, love, frustration, and hope. These stories matter because they represent real human experiences that deserve recognition and support. Too often, partners find themselves isolated, questioning their perceptions, and wondering if they're the problem.

The medical community focuses primarily on treating the person with the disorder, which makes sense from a clinical perspective. But this approach often overlooks the partners who experience secondary trauma, develop anxiety disorders, struggle with codependency, and sometimes lose their sense of identity in the process of trying to maintain these challenging relationships.

Your experience as a partner has validity regardless of your partner's specific diagnosis or your relationship outcome. You might have stayed and found strategies that work. You might have left to protect your mental health. You might currently be weighing difficult decisions about your future. All of these experiences deserve acknowledgment and support.

Case Example 2: David's Journey with Dependent Personality Disorder David married Sarah when they were both 25. At first, he felt flattered by her need for his input on every decision, from what to wear to work to which grocery store to visit. Her dependence on him felt like love and trust. But over time, the constant need for reassurance and decision-making became overwhelming.

Sarah couldn't make any choice without David's approval. She would call him multiple times during his workday to ask about minor decisions. When he traveled for business, Sarah would experience panic attacks and beg him not to leave. Friends started avoiding them because Sarah couldn't participate in conversations without constantly checking David's reactions.

David felt trapped between his love for Sarah and his need for autonomy. Well-meaning friends suggested he was "lucky to have someone who valued his opinion so much," but they didn't understand the exhausting responsibility of being another person's sole decision-maker. When David finally learned about dependent personality disorder, he realized that Sarah's behavior wasn't about love—it was about a deep-seated fear of making decisions and taking responsibility for her own life.

Beyond BPD

Why Comprehensive Coverage Changes Everything

Walk into any bookstore's self-help section, and you'll find dozens of books about borderline personality disorder relationships. "Stop Walking on Eggshells" has sold over a million copies, creating an entire industry around BPD relationship guidance. But what if your partner has narcissistic personality disorder, avoidant personality disorder, or obsessive-compulsive personality disorder? The resources dwindle to almost nothing.

This gap in available information creates several problems. First, partners dealing with other personality disorders feel isolated and unsupported. Second, they may misinterpret their partner's behavior through a BPD lens when different dynamics are at play. Third, they miss out on disorder-specific strategies that could improve their relationship or help them make informed decisions about their future.

Each personality disorder creates distinct challenges and requires different approaches. The communication strategies that work with someone who has avoidant personality disorder might be counterproductive with someone who has histrionic personality disorder. The boundary-setting techniques effective for narcissistic relationships could be harmful in dependent personality disorder situations.

Case Example 3: Jennifer's Misdiagnosis Confusion Jennifer's husband Mark exhibited many concerning behaviors: emotional detachment, preference for solitude, and difficulty expressing affection. When Jennifer researched their relationship problems online, most resources pointed to either autism spectrum disorders or borderline personality disorder. Neither seemed to fit completely.

Mark wasn't prone to emotional outbursts like BPD descriptions suggested, nor did he show the social communication challenges associated with autism. Instead, he seemed to have a fundamental lack of interest in close relationships, including their marriage. He preferred solitary activities, showed little emotional range, and seemed indifferent to Jennifer's feelings.

When Jennifer finally found information about schizoid personality disorder, everything clicked into place. Mark's behavior wasn't about not loving her—it was about a pervasive pattern of detachment from social relationships and restricted emotional expression. This understanding changed Jennifer's approach entirely. Instead of trying to create more emotional intimacy (which only made Mark withdraw further), she learned to appreciate the subtle ways he showed care and to build a relationship that accommodated both their needs.

How to Use This Book

Finding Your Path Through Confusion to Clarity

This book is designed as both a reference guide and a step-by-step roadmap. You don't need to read it cover to cover (although you certainly can). Instead, you can focus on the sections most relevant to your situation.

The structure moves from general understanding to specific disorders to practical strategies. Part I helps you understand personality disorders broadly and examine your own role in the relationship dynamic. Parts II, III, and IV cover each personality disorder in detail, with real stories and practical strategies. Part V focuses on moving forward, making decisions, and healing.

Each chapter includes specific tools you can use immediately:

- Communication scripts for difficult conversations
- Safety assessment guidelines when needed

- Self-care strategies to protect your mental health

- Decision-making frameworks for complex situations

- Hope stories from others who've navigated similar challenges

Use the index to find specific topics quickly. If you're in crisis, go directly to the safety planning sections. If you're trying to understand your partner's behavior, start with the disorder-specific chapters. If you're considering leaving the relationship, focus on the decision-making chapters.

Success Stories Exist for Every Disorder

One of the most important messages in this book is that hope exists for every personality disorder, though success might look different than you initially imagined. Some couples find ways to build satisfying relationships by understanding the disorder and adapting their expectations and strategies. Others find peace by ending relationships that were fundamentally incompatible with their needs and values.

Success isn't measured by staying together or breaking up. Success is measured by your ability to make informed decisions, protect your mental health, maintain your sense of identity, and create a life that aligns with your values and needs.

Research shows that many personality disorders can improve with appropriate treatment, though change typically happens slowly and requires the person with the disorder to be motivated and engaged in the process. Partners can't create this change, but they can create conditions that either support or hinder progress.

Every personality disorder chapter in this book includes examples of relationships that found stability and satisfaction. These aren't fairy tale endings where everything becomes easy, but realistic examples of how understanding, appropriate strategies, and sometimes professional help can create positive outcomes.

Reality of Change

Change in personality disorder relationships requires realistic expectations. These disorders develop over many years, often starting in childhood, and involve deeply ingrained patterns of thinking, feeling, and behaving. Quick fixes don't exist, and love alone isn't enough to create change.

However, improvement is possible when the person with the disorder recognizes the impact of their behavior and commits to treatment. Dialectical Behavior Therapy (DBT), Cognitive Behavioral Therapy (CBT), and other evidence-based treatments can help people with personality disorders develop better emotional regulation, communication skills, and relationship patterns.

Your role as a partner involves understanding what you can and cannot control, developing your own coping strategies, and making decisions about what you're willing and able to handle in the relationship.

Building Your Support Network

Reading this book is an important first step, but it shouldn't be your only source of support. Consider building a network that might include:

- Individual therapy with someone experienced in personality disorders

- Support groups for partners (online or in-person)

- Trusted friends who can provide perspective and emotional support

- Family members who understand your situation

- Professional resources like employee assistance programs

Isolation makes everything harder. Connection and support make difficult situations more manageable and help you maintain perspective during challenging times.

Looking Ahead Together

This book will take you through a journey of understanding, from the basics of personality disorders to specific strategies for each type, to making decisions about your future. You'll read real stories from people who've faced similar challenges and discover practical tools that can improve your situation.

Each chapter builds on the previous ones, creating a foundation of knowledge and skills you can use regardless of what decisions you make about your relationship. By the end, you'll have a clear understanding of personality disorders, your own patterns and needs, and the tools to create positive change in your life.

The path ahead may not be easy, but you don't have to walk it alone. Millions of people have faced similar challenges, and many have found ways to create lives they love. Your story matters, your experience is valid, and hope exists for your future.

Key Takeaways

- Personality disorders affect 10-15% of adults, making them more common than many physical health conditions

- Partners of people with personality disorders face unique challenges that require specific understanding and strategies

- Each personality disorder creates different dynamics and requires different approaches

- Success in these relationships can take many forms, from finding stability together to making healthy decisions to separate

- Change is possible but requires realistic expectations, professional support, and time

- You deserve support, understanding, and the tools to make informed decisions about your life

Chapter 2: What Your Partner Can't Tell You

The late-night conversations often go in circles. Your partner knows something feels wrong in their relationships, but they can't articulate what or why. They might say things like "I don't know why I react this way" or "I can't help it." These aren't excuses or manipulation tactics—they're often genuine expressions of confusion about their own internal experiences. Understanding how personality disorders develop and function can transform your perspective on these confusing moments.

Personality Disorder Brain

Personality disorders represent fundamental differences in how someone's brain processes emotions, relationships, and self-identity. These aren't temporary states or choices—they're pervasive patterns that affect virtually every aspect of a person's life. To understand this, imagine personality as the operating system of human psychology. Most people have relatively stable, flexible operating systems that adapt to different situations while maintaining core functionality. Personality disorders are like operating systems with specific glitches or programming differences that consistently affect how information gets processed.

The brain research shows fascinating differences in people with personality disorders. Neuroimaging studies reveal altered activity in areas responsible for emotional regulation, impulse control, and social cognition. For example, people with borderline personality disorder often show decreased activity in the prefrontal cortex (the brain's "CEO" responsible for decision-making and impulse control) and increased activity in the amygdala (the alarm system that triggers fight-or-flight responses).

These brain differences aren't defects or damage—they're variations that create predictable patterns of thinking and behaving. Understanding this helps explain why logical arguments often don't change your partner's reactions and why they might struggle to control responses that seem obviously counterproductive to you.

Case Example 1: Understanding Tom's Explosive Reactions Sarah lived with Tom for five years, constantly confused by his explosive reactions to minor stressors. When Sarah would suggest they needed to leave for an appointment in ten minutes, Tom would suddenly become agitated, start yelling about feeling controlled, and sometimes storm out of the house entirely. Sarah tried everything—giving more notice, asking instead of stating, even handling all the scheduling herself.

Nothing worked because Sarah was trying to solve a logical problem with logical solutions. But Tom's brain processed Sarah's reminders as threats to his autonomy, triggering his fight-or-flight system. His angry reactions weren't about the appointments—they were about his brain's tendency to interpret normal relationship interactions as attempts to control or diminish him.

When Sarah learned about narcissistic personality disorder, she realized that Tom's brain consistently misinterpreted neutral interactions as attacks on his self-esteem. This understanding didn't excuse his behavior, but it helped Sarah stop taking his reactions personally and develop strategies that worked with his brain patterns instead of against them.

Why Love Isn't Enough

The Neuroscience of Ingrained Patterns

One of the most painful realizations for partners is that love, patience, and understanding—while valuable—aren't sufficient to change personality disorder patterns. These patterns exist at a neurological level and involve automatic responses that bypass conscious decision-making. It's similar to trying to stop a reflex by thinking about it—the reaction happens before conscious thought can intervene.

The neuroscience research reveals that personality disorders involve differences in several key brain systems:

Emotional Processing Systems: Many personality disorders involve difficulties with emotional regulation. The brain either overreacts or underreacts to emotional stimuli, creating patterns of emotional instability or emotional numbing.

Social Cognition Networks: These are the brain systems responsible for understanding others' thoughts, feelings, and intentions. When these systems function differently, it affects how someone interprets social interactions and relationship dynamics.

Self-Awareness Circuits: Some personality disorders involve limited insight into one's own behavior and its impact on others. This isn't about intelligence—it's about specific brain functions that support self-reflection and awareness.

Attachment Systems: The brain networks that govern how we form and maintain close relationships can function differently in personality disorders, creating patterns of either desperate clinging or defensive distancing.

Understanding these brain differences helps explain why personality disorder behaviors are so consistent and why they don't change simply because someone wants them to or recognizes they're problematic.

Case Example 2: Linda's Attachment Confusion Linda's girlfriend Maria had a pattern that seemed impossible to understand. Maria would become intensely attached very quickly, wanting to spend all their time together and talking about moving in together after just a few weeks of dating. But then, seemingly without warning, Maria would become distant and critical, finding fault with everything Linda did.

This push-pull pattern repeated in cycles that left Linda emotionally exhausted and constantly anxious about which version of Maria she would encounter each day. Linda assumed that if Maria really loved her, she would stop these hurtful patterns. But Maria's behavior wasn't about her feelings for Linda—it was about her brain's attachment system, which had learned early in life that closeness leads to abandonment.

Maria's brain would trigger intense bonding feelings initially (the push phase), but then her fear-based neural networks would activate, interpreting normal relationship closeness as dangerous vulnerability (the pull phase). Maria couldn't simply decide to stop this pattern because it operated at a level below conscious choice.

Attachment Theory

How Childhood Shapes Adult Relationships

Attachment theory provides the foundation for understanding how personality disorders develop and persist. Research by Psychiatry Online and numerous other sources shows that early childhood experiences literally shape brain development, particularly in areas responsible for emotional regulation and relationship formation.

Children develop internal working models of relationships based on their early experiences with caregivers. These models become templates that guide expectations and behaviors in future relationships. In healthy development, children learn that relationships are generally safe, predictable, and rewarding. They develop secure attachment patterns that allow them to trust others while maintaining their own sense of identity.

But when children experience inconsistent caregiving, trauma, neglect, or other adverse experiences, they develop insecure attachment patterns as survival strategies. These patterns might include:

Anxious Attachment: Becoming hypervigilant about signs of rejection or abandonment, leading to clingy or demanding behavior in relationships.

Avoidant Attachment: Learning that emotional needs won't be met consistently, leading to excessive self-reliance and emotional distance in relationships.

Disorganized Attachment: Experiencing caregivers as both sources of comfort and danger, leading to chaotic relationship patterns that swing between extremes.

These attachment patterns become encoded in the developing brain and continue influencing relationship behavior throughout life. Personality disorders often represent extreme versions of insecure attachment patterns that persist into adulthood.

Case Example 3: Understanding Jake's Avoidance Rebecca married Jake after a two-year courtship where he seemed emotionally available and connected. But after marriage, Jake became increasingly distant and seemed to panic whenever Rebecca wanted to discuss their relationship or future plans. He would change the subject, leave the room, or become irritable when Rebecca tried to create emotional intimacy.

Rebecca initially thought Jake was losing interest in their marriage or having an affair. But when she learned about Jake's childhood experiences, a different picture emerged. Jake's mother had severe depression and would alternate between emotional neediness and complete withdrawal. As a child, Jake learned that emotional closeness with important people led to overwhelming demands he couldn't meet and abandonment he couldn't prevent.

Jake's adult brain still carried these early templates. When Rebecca wanted emotional closeness, Jake's attachment system interpreted this as dangerous territory that would lead to overwhelming demands or eventual abandonment. His withdrawal wasn't about not loving Rebecca—it was about his brain's learned strategy for protecting himself from what it perceived as relationship threats.

The Difference Between "Difficult" and Disordered

Many people have difficult personality traits or go through challenging periods in relationships. The key difference with personality disorders lies in pervasiveness, persistence, and impact. Personality disorders involve patterns that:

- Appear across multiple areas of life, not just romantic relationships

- Remain consistent over time, typically beginning in early adulthood or adolescence

- Cause significant distress or impairment in social, occupational, or other important functioning

- Are inflexible and difficult to change even when they create obvious problems

Everyone has bad days, reacts poorly to stress, or struggles with certain relationship dynamics. But personality disorders involve patterns that persist regardless of circumstances and resist change even when the consequences are severe.

The diagnostic criteria require that these patterns be stable across time and situations. Someone might act jealous and controlling during a period of high stress but return to normal functioning once the stress passes. In contrast, someone with paranoid personality disorder will show persistent distrust and suspicion across various relationships and circumstances.

Understanding this distinction helps partners recognize when they're dealing with temporary relationship problems versus fundamental personality patterns that require different approaches and expectations.

Common Myths That Keep Partners Stuck

Several myths about personality disorders persist in popular culture and even among some mental health professionals. These myths can trap partners in ineffective strategies and unrealistic expectations.

Myth 1: "People with personality disorders can't change" While personality disorders are persistent and challenging to treat, research shows that many people can learn better coping strategies and develop healthier relationship patterns with appropriate treatment and motivation. Change is possible but typically requires professional help and occurs gradually over years.

Myth 2: "Love will heal them" This romantic notion keeps many partners trapped in cycles of trying harder to provide enough love, understanding, or support to fix their partner's mental health. While love and support are valuable, personality disorders require professional treatment and the person's own commitment to change.

Myth 3: "They're just manipulative" Many personality disorder behaviors look manipulative from the outside, but they're often desperate attempts to manage overwhelming emotions or meet fundamental psychological needs. Understanding the underlying emotional state doesn't excuse harmful behavior, but it can inform more effective responses.

Myth 4: "If they really loved me, they would change" This myth confuses love with the ability to change deeply ingrained psychological patterns. Someone can genuinely love their partner while still being unable to control personality disorder symptoms without professional help and significant effort.

Myth 5: "I can fix this if I just find the right approach" This keeps partners stuck in endless cycles of trying new strategies to manage their partner's symptoms. While partners can learn more effective ways to respond, they cannot cure or control another person's personality disorder.

Recognizing the Impact on Your Own Mental Health

Living with someone who has a personality disorder often creates secondary effects on partners' mental health. Common impacts include:

Anxiety Disorders: Constantly walking on eggshells or trying to predict and prevent emotional outbursts can create chronic anxiety.

Depression: The emotional exhaustion and sense of hopelessness that often accompany these relationships can lead to depressive symptoms.

Trauma Responses: Some partners develop symptoms similar to post-traumatic stress disorder, particularly if they've experienced emotional, psychological, or physical abuse.

Codependency: The tendency to become overly focused on managing another person's emotions and behaviors at the expense of your own well-being.

Identity Issues: Long-term exposure to gaslighting, criticism, or emotional instability can erode your sense of self and confidence in your own perceptions.

Recognizing these impacts is crucial for several reasons. First, it validates your experience and helps you understand that your struggles are normal responses to abnormal situations. Second, it highlights the importance of protecting and caring for your own mental health. Third, it can inform decisions about what level of dysfunction you can sustainably handle in a relationship.

Taking Care of Yourself First

Understanding personality disorders is important, but it's equally important to understand your own needs, limits, and well-being. You cannot help anyone else from a place of depletion and poor mental health. Taking care of yourself isn't selfish—it's necessary for making good decisions and maintaining the emotional resources needed for any relationship, but especially challenging ones.

Self-care in personality disorder relationships goes beyond bubble baths and exercise. It involves setting and maintaining boundaries, getting professional support when needed, maintaining connections with friends and family, and regularly assessing whether the relationship is compatible with your mental health and life goals.

Key Takeaways

- Personality disorders involve brain differences that create consistent patterns of thinking, feeling, and behaving

- These patterns develop early in life and operate largely outside conscious control

- Love, patience, and understanding—while valuable—are not sufficient to change personality disorder patterns

- Attachment theory helps explain how early experiences shape adult relationship patterns

- Personality disorders differ from temporary difficulties in their pervasiveness, persistence, and impact

- Common myths about personality disorders can trap partners in ineffective strategies

- Partners often experience secondary mental health impacts that require attention and care

Chapter 3: Recognizing Yourself - The Partner's Journey

Standing in front of the bathroom mirror at 3 AM, you might catch a glimpse of someone you barely recognize. The person staring back has developed skills you never thought you'd need—reading micro-expressions for signs of impending emotional storms, crafting careful responses to avoid triggering explosive reactions, managing complex logistics to prevent crises. You've become an expert in someone else's emotional weather patterns, but somewhere along the way, you lost touch with your own internal compass.

The Caregiver Trap

When Helping Becomes Harmful

The transformation happens gradually, almost imperceptibly. It starts with natural impulses to help someone you love who's struggling. You notice patterns—certain situations trigger your partner's distress, specific words or actions seem to escalate conflicts, particular approaches help calm intense emotions. Your caring nature leads you to adjust your behavior to minimize their distress and maximize their stability.

Initially, this feels like love in action. You're being supportive, understanding, accommodating. But over time, these helpful adjustments expand and solidify into a complex system where your entire life revolves around managing another person's emotional state. You stop making plans that might upset them, avoid topics that trigger reactions, and constantly monitor their moods to anticipate needs and prevent problems.

According to research from Royal Life Detox and other treatment centers, this pattern—known as caregiver syndrome or caregiver burnout—is extremely common among partners of people with personality disorders. The helper gradually assumes responsibility for the emotional well-being of another adult, often at the expense of their own needs, goals, and mental health.

Case Example 1: Michelle's Vanishing Act Michelle met David when they were both 28. David had been diagnosed with borderline personality disorder, but Michelle didn't fully understand what that meant. She knew he had been in therapy and took medication, and she admired his openness about his mental health struggles.

In the beginning, Michelle's support seemed to help David tremendously. When he felt overwhelmed at work, she would listen for hours and help him process his emotions. When he struggled with social anxiety, she would accompany him to events and help facilitate conversations. When he had conflicts with friends or family, she would offer perspectives and help him draft careful text messages.

Two years into their relationship, Michelle realized she hadn't seen her own friends in months. She had stopped pursuing hobbies because they took time away from supporting David. She had turned down a promotion that would require occasional travel because David couldn't handle her being away. Her entire identity had become "David's supportive girlfriend," and she couldn't remember what her own interests and goals had been.

The most concerning part was that David wasn't improving despite all her support. If anything, he seemed more dependent on her emotional management and less capable of handling challenges independently. Michelle had become an enabler rather than a support system.

Codependency Patterns Before They Take Root

Codependency represents a dysfunctional relationship pattern where one person becomes excessively focused on caring for another person's emotional needs while neglecting their own well-being. Wikipedia and Positive Psychology research identify several key characteristics of codependent relationships:

Excessive Caretaking: Taking responsibility for another adult's emotions, decisions, and consequences. This goes beyond normal support and involves assuming roles that should belong to the other person.

Difficulty Setting Boundaries: Struggling to say no to requests for help, even when those requests are unreasonable or harmful to your own well-being.

Identity Fusion: Your sense of self becomes intertwined with the other person's emotional state. You feel good when they feel good, and you feel responsible when they struggle.

Enabling Behaviors: Actions that inadvertently prevent the other person from facing natural consequences of their choices, thus preventing growth and learning.

Neglecting Self-Care: Consistently prioritizing the other person's needs over your own basic requirements for physical and mental health.

Loss of Personal Interests: Gradually abandoning your own hobbies, friendships, goals, and activities in service of the relationship.

The tricky aspect of codependency in personality disorder relationships is that many of these patterns can initially appear healthy and loving. The key difference lies in balance and sustainability. Healthy relationships involve mutual support where both people maintain their individual identities, interests, and responsibilities.

Case Example 2: Robert's Financial Rescue Mission Robert's wife Amanda had narcissistic personality disorder, though she was never officially diagnosed. Amanda had a pattern of starting grand business ventures with enormous enthusiasm, only to abandon them when they required sustained effort or when she encountered criticism. Each failure would trigger intense shame and depression, during which Amanda would become suicidal and blame Robert for not being supportive enough.

Over their eight-year marriage, Robert had funded seven different business attempts, totaling nearly $80,000 from their savings and retirement accounts. Each time Amanda would promise this venture would be different, and each time Robert would agree to help because he feared what might happen if he said no.

Robert told himself he was being a supportive husband, but his pattern of financial rescue was actually preventing Amanda from facing the consequences of her choices and learning more realistic goal-setting. Meanwhile, Robert was developing anxiety about their financial future and resentment about Amanda's lack of follow-through, though he felt too guilty to express these feelings.

When Robert finally set a boundary—no more business funding until Amanda completed a business planning course and demonstrated sustained effort on a smaller project—Amanda accused him of trying to sabotage her dreams. But the boundary forced Amanda to confront her pattern of unrealistic expectations and poor follow-through, ultimately leading her to seek therapy.

Your Attachment Style and Why It Matters

Your own attachment style—the patterns you learned in childhood about how relationships work—significantly influences how you respond to a partner with a personality disorder. Understanding your attachment style helps explain why you might be drawn to certain relationship dynamics and why some situations feel particularly triggering or compelling.

Secure Attachment (about 50-60% of adults): You generally feel comfortable with intimacy and independence. You can maintain your sense of self in relationships while also being emotionally available to partners. If you have secure attachment, you might be drawn to help someone with a personality disorder because you believe relationships can be healing, but you're also likely to recognize when dynamics become unhealthy.

Anxious Attachment (about 15-20% of adults): You tend to worry about your partner's feelings toward you and may become preoccupied with the relationship. You might interpret your partner's personality disorder symptoms as signs that they're losing interest or that you need to try harder to maintain the connection. This can lead to increased caretaking and difficulty setting boundaries.

Avoidant Attachment (about 20-25% of adults): You tend to value independence and may feel uncomfortable with too much closeness. Paradoxically, you might find yourself drawn to partners with personality disorders because their emotional intensity creates the distance you're comfortable with, even as it creates other problems.

Disorganized Attachment (about 5-10% of adults): You might have conflicting desires for closeness and distance, often stemming from childhood experiences with caregivers who were both comforting and frightening. This can create a complex dynamic with personality disorder partners where you're simultaneously drawn to and overwhelmed by their emotional intensity.

Case Example 3: Lisa's Anxious Attachment Trap Lisa had anxious attachment patterns stemming from childhood experiences with an emotionally unpredictable mother. When she met Jake, who had avoidant personality disorder, she initially felt intrigued by his mysterious, hard-to-read nature. Jake's emotional unavailability triggered Lisa's anxiety, which she interpreted as intense romantic feelings.

Jake's tendency to withdraw when Lisa wanted closeness activated all of Lisa's abandonment fears. She responded by trying harder to connect, which made Jake feel suffocated and withdraw further. Lisa interpreted Jake's withdrawal as confirmation that she wasn't loveable enough, so she would increase her efforts to be the perfect girlfriend.

This created a cycle where Lisa's anxious pursuit triggered Jake's avoidant withdrawal, which triggered more anxious pursuit from Lisa. Both partners were trapped in their attachment patterns, each inadvertently triggering the other's deepest fears. Lisa felt constantly rejected and anxious, while Jake felt constantly pressured and suffocated.

Understanding attachment styles helped Lisa recognize that her intense feelings weren't necessarily about love—they were about her anxiety system being activated. She learned to distinguish between genuine compatibility and attachment system activation, which helped her make better decisions about relationships.

The "Fixer" Mindset and Its Dangers

Many partners of people with personality disorders have what psychologists call a "fixer" mentality—the belief that with enough love, understanding, patience, or the right approach, they can help their partner overcome their mental health challenges. This mindset often stems from positive qualities like compassion, optimism, and problem-solving skills, but it can become problematic in personality disorder relationships.

The fixer mindset creates several problems:

Unrealistic Responsibility: You begin to believe that your partner's emotional stability depends on your actions, which creates enormous pressure and guilt when they struggle.

Boundary Erosion: The focus on fixing the other person often involves accepting behaviors and treatment that you wouldn't tolerate in other relationships.

Identity Loss: Your sense of purpose and value becomes tied to your success in helping your partner, rather than your own goals and accomplishments.

Enabling: Your attempts to prevent your partner's distress may actually prevent them from developing their own coping skills and seeking appropriate professional help.

Resentment: When your fixing attempts don't work (as they often don't), you may develop resentment toward your partner for not appreciating your efforts or not getting better despite your help.

The reality is that personality disorders require professional treatment and the person's own commitment to change. While partners can provide support and learn more effective ways to respond, they cannot cure or control another person's mental health condition.

Building Your Emotional First-Aid Kit

Living with someone who has a personality disorder requires developing specific emotional skills and resources to protect your own mental health. Think of this as building an emotional first-aid kit—tools and strategies you can use quickly when situations become overwhelming.

Grounding Techniques: Methods to stay connected to your own reality and emotional state when interactions become confusing or intense. This might include:

- Deep breathing exercises you can do anywhere
- Physical grounding (noticing what you can see, hear, touch around you)

26

- Positive self-talk phrases that remind you of your worth and perspective

- Quick body scans to check in with your own emotional state

Communication Strategies: Scripts and approaches that can de-escalate conflicts and protect your emotional boundaries:

- "I" statements that express your needs without attacking your partner

- Broken record technique for maintaining boundaries despite pressure

- Ways to disengage from circular arguments

- Phrases that validate your partner's feelings without accepting blame

Support Systems: Relationships and resources outside your primary relationship that provide perspective and emotional support:

- Individual therapy with someone experienced in personality disorders

- Support groups for partners (online or in-person)

- Trusted friends who can provide reality checks and emotional support

- Family members who understand your situation

- Professional resources like employee assistance programs

Self-Care Practices: Activities and practices that help you maintain your own emotional and physical well-being:

- Regular exercise or movement that helps process stress

- Hobbies and interests that connect you to your own identity

- Spiritual or mindfulness practices that provide perspective

- Adequate sleep, nutrition, and medical care

- Time in nature or other environments that restore your energy

Safety Planning: Strategies for situations that might become dangerous or overwhelming:

- Safe places you can go if you need space

- People you can call for support in crisis situations

- Important documents and resources kept accessible

- Clear criteria for when to seek professional help

- Plans for protecting children if they're involved

Recognizing Your Own Growth and Healing Needs

Relationships with personality disorder dynamics often create secondary trauma in partners. You might develop symptoms similar to anxiety disorders, depression, or even post-traumatic stress. These aren't signs of weakness—they're normal responses to abnormal levels of stress and emotional chaos.

Common experiences include:

- Hypervigilance (constantly monitoring your partner's mood and reactions)

- Anxiety about normal relationship interactions

- Difficulty trusting your own perceptions (especially if you've experienced gaslighting)

- Emotional numbing or feeling disconnected from your own emotions

- Sleep problems, appetite changes, or other physical symptoms of chronic stress

- Difficulty enjoying activities that used to bring you pleasure

- Social isolation or difficulty maintaining other relationships

Recognizing these impacts is important for several reasons. First, it validates your experience and helps you understand that your struggles are normal responses to challenging circumstances. Second, it highlights the importance of getting support for your own healing, regardless of what happens in your relationship. Third, it can inform decisions about what you can sustainably handle and what changes need to happen for your own well-being.

The Path to Healthy Choices

Understanding your own patterns, needs, and healing requirements is essential for making healthy decisions about your relationship. You cannot make good choices from a place of depletion, confusion, or fear. Taking time to understand your own psychology and attachment patterns isn't selfish—it's necessary for both your well-being and for any positive changes that might be possible in your relationship.

The goal isn't to become a perfect partner who never triggers your loved one's symptoms. The goal is to become a healthy person who can engage in relationships from a place of strength, clarity, and self-respect. This might mean learning to support your partner in healthier ways, or it might mean recognizing that the relationship isn't sustainable for your mental health. Either outcome is valid when it comes from a place of self-awareness and genuine choice rather than fear or obligation.

Key Takeaways

- The caregiver trap involves gradually assuming responsibility for another adult's emotional well-being at the expense of your own needs

- Codependency patterns often develop slowly and can initially appear to be loving and supportive behaviors

- Your attachment style influences how you respond to personality disorder dynamics and what situations feel particularly triggering

- The "fixer" mindset, while stemming from positive qualities, can create unrealistic expectations and prevent healthy boundaries

- Building an emotional first-aid kit with grounding techniques, communication strategies, and support systems is essential for maintaining mental health

- Partners often experience secondary trauma that requires recognition and healing, regardless of relationship outcomes

- Self-awareness and understanding your own patterns is necessary for making healthy decisions about your relationship future

Chapter 4: Paranoid Personality Disorder

When Trust Becomes Impossible

The accusation comes out of nowhere, hitting you like cold water. Your partner found a receipt from lunch with a colleague and has constructed an elaborate theory about your affair, complete with detailed timelines and evidence that makes no sense to anyone but them. No amount of explanation satisfies their suspicion. Your truthful answers become proof that you're a skilled liar. Your emotional responses become evidence of your guilt. You're trapped in a system where innocence cannot be proven and trust cannot be rebuilt.

The Reality of Paranoid Jealousy

Paranoid personality disorder transforms ordinary relationships into high-stakes investigations where you are always the primary suspect. Your partner's brain has developed a hyperactive threat-detection system that interprets neutral interactions as potential dangers and innocent behaviors as evidence of betrayal or deception.

This isn't the occasional jealousy that many couples experience. Paranoid personality disorder involves pervasive distrust that affects virtually every aspect of the relationship. Your partner might:

- Monitor your communications, demanding to read texts, emails, and social media

- Question your whereabouts with detailed cross-examinations

- Interpret friendly interactions with others as romantic or threatening

31

- Remember and catalog minor inconsistencies in your stories as proof of deception

- Become suspicious of your family and friends, seeing them as threats to the relationship

- Feel threatened by your professional success or independent activities

The surveillance often extends beyond romantic jealousy to include suspicion about your motives, your loyalty, and your basic honesty about everyday matters. You might find yourself being questioned about why you chose a particular route home, why you spoke to a neighbor, or why you seemed distracted during dinner.

Case Example 1: Sarah's Ten-Year Investigation Sarah married Robert when they were both in their late twenties. In the early months of their relationship, Robert's attentiveness felt flattering. He wanted to know about her day, her thoughts, her feelings. He seemed fascinated by every detail of her life. Sarah interpreted this as intense love and interest.

Gradually, the questions became interrogations. Robert would ask about conversations Sarah had with coworkers, then ask again later to see if her story remained consistent. He would drive by her workplace to "surprise her with lunch" but was actually checking to see if her car was really there. He installed tracking software on her phone "for safety" but used it to monitor her every movement.

When Sarah got a promotion that required occasional travel, Robert became convinced she was having affairs in different cities. He would call her hotel rooms multiple times per night, demand photos of her room and meals to prove she was alone, and become enraged if she didn't answer immediately. Sarah's work began to suffer because she spent so much energy managing Robert's suspicions.

The most heartbreaking part was that Robert's distrust wasn't based on any actual betrayal. Sarah had never cheated, lied about her whereabouts, or given Robert any reason to doubt her faithfulness. But his paranoid personality disorder created a lens through which all of Sarah's innocent actions appeared suspicious. Ten years into their marriage, Robert was more convinced than ever that Sarah was deceiving him, despite having no evidence beyond his own distorted interpretations.

"I Love You But I Don't Believe You"

Understanding the Paranoid Mindset

One of the most confusing aspects of paranoid personality disorder is that your partner can genuinely love you while simultaneously believing you're capable of elaborate deceptions. This isn't a contradiction—it reflects the complex nature of paranoid thinking patterns.

People with paranoid personality disorder often have a split view of relationships. They desperately want connection and love, but they also believe that people are fundamentally untrustworthy and motivated by hidden agendas. This creates a painful internal conflict where they love you and want to trust you, but their paranoid thought patterns make trust feel impossible and dangerous.

The paranoid mindset involves several key characteristics:

Hypervigilance: Constant scanning for signs of threat, betrayal, or deception. This creates exhaustion for both partners—the paranoid person is always "on guard," and you feel like you're always under scrutiny.

Confirmation Bias: The tendency to interpret ambiguous information as confirming their suspicions while dismissing or explaining away evidence that contradicts their fears.

Attribution Errors: Assuming that neutral or positive actions have negative motivations. For example, your kindness might be interpreted as guilt, or your attempt to reassure them might be seen as manipulation.

Memory Distortions: Remembering events in ways that support their paranoid beliefs while forgetting or minimizing contradictory information.

Projection: Attributing their own thoughts or feelings to others. If they're feeling angry, they might assume you're plotting against them.

Understanding these patterns helps explain why logical arguments and evidence don't resolve paranoid suspicions. Your partner's brain is operating from a different set of assumptions about how relationships work and what motivates people's behavior.

Practical Strategies for the "Walking on Eggshells" Partner

Living with paranoid personality disorder requires specific strategies that account for your partner's unique psychological patterns. Traditional relationship advice—like "just communicate better" or "be more understanding"—often backfires in paranoid relationships because it doesn't address the underlying thought patterns driving the behavior.

Consistency is Crucial: Maintain extremely consistent patterns in your behavior, communication, and routines. While this might feel restrictive, it reduces the number of variables your partner's paranoid mind can interpret as suspicious.

Document Reality: Keep records of important conversations, decisions, and events. This isn't about proving your innocence—it's about having objective information when your partner's memory distorts events to support their suspicions.

Avoid Defensive Responses: When accused, resist the urge to become emotional or defensive, as these responses will be interpreted as proof of guilt. Instead, acknowledge their feelings while calmly stating facts.

Set Clear Boundaries: Establish limits on surveillance behaviors that you can maintain consistently. For example, you might agree to share your location but not to detailed interrogations about every interaction.

Don't Enable Paranoid Behaviors: While you can provide reasonable reassurance, don't participate in elaborate efforts to "prove" your innocence, as this typically escalates rather than resolves paranoid concerns.

Case Example 2: Managing Daily Paranoid Episodes Jennifer learned to navigate her husband Mark's paranoid personality disorder by developing a consistent daily routine that minimized triggers while protecting her own mental health. Mark would become suspicious if Jennifer's routine varied in any way, interpreting changes as evidence that she was hiding something.

Jennifer established clear patterns: she would text Mark when she arrived at work, during lunch, and when she left for home. She would call him on her drive home and let him know if she needed to stop anywhere. She kept receipts for all purchases and maintained consistent explanations for any routine changes.

This might sound oppressive, but Jennifer found that consistency actually gave her more freedom than the constant interrogations that occurred when Mark felt uncertain about her activities. The key was that Jennifer chose these boundaries rather than having them imposed through conflict and accusations.

Jennifer also set limits on Mark's surveillance behaviors. She agreed to share her phone location but refused to hand over her phone for inspection. She would answer reasonable questions about her day but wouldn't participate in detailed cross-examinations about her conversations or interactions.

Most importantly, Jennifer maintained her own support system and refused to isolate herself despite Mark's suspicions about her friends and family. She would inform Mark about social plans rather than asking permission, and she would go regardless of his paranoid concerns about her friends' motivations.

Safety Planning When Suspicion Turns Dangerous

Paranoid personality disorder can escalate into dangerous territory when suspicions become so intense that your partner believes you pose a genuine threat to them or when they decide to take action to "protect" themselves from your perceived betrayal. Safety planning becomes crucial when paranoid thoughts lead to:

- Threats of violence based on imagined betrayals

- Attempts to isolate you from all outside relationships

- Extreme surveillance that interferes with your work or daily functioning

- Destruction of your property or belongings as "punishment" for imagined wrongs

- Involvement of others in monitoring or controlling your behavior

- Threats to harm themselves if you leave or if their suspicions are confirmed

Creating a Safety Plan:

Identify Warning Signs: Learn to recognize when your partner's paranoid thoughts are escalating toward dangerous territory. This might include increased agitation, making specific threats, or beginning to involve others in their suspicions.

Establish Safe Contacts: Maintain relationships with people your partner doesn't monitor or control. Have safe people you can contact quickly if situations escalate.

Secure Important Documents: Keep copies of identification, financial documents, and other important papers in a secure location your partner cannot access.

Plan Safe Locations: Identify places you can go quickly if you need to leave, including friends' homes, family members, or shelters if necessary.

Financial Safety: Maintain access to funds that your partner cannot control or monitor if possible.

Professional Resources: Have contact information for domestic violence hotlines, mental health crisis services, and legal resources readily available.

Can This Relationship Be Saved?

Deciding whether to continue a relationship with someone who has paranoid personality disorder requires honest assessment of several factors. Unlike some other personality disorders where improvement is common with treatment, paranoid personality disorder is particularly challenging because people with this condition rarely seek help voluntarily and often don't believe they have a problem.

Factors that Suggest Hope for Improvement:

- Your partner occasionally recognizes that their suspicions might be excessive or unrealistic

- They're willing to discuss their paranoid thoughts rather than simply acting on them

- They can sometimes accept reassurance, even if it doesn't last long

- They're willing to seek therapy or consider that their thought patterns might be problematic

- The paranoid behaviors haven't escalated to dangerous or severely controlling levels

- You can maintain some independence and outside relationships

- There are periods of relative calm between paranoid episodes

Factors that Suggest the Relationship May Not Be Sustainable:

- Your partner is completely convinced that their suspicions are justified and shows no insight into their paranoid thinking

- The paranoid behaviors are escalating in frequency or intensity

- You've lost your independence, career opportunities, or important relationships due to their suspicions

- You feel unsafe or fear for your physical safety

- Your mental health is severely impacted by the constant suspicion and surveillance

- Children are being affected by the paranoid atmosphere in the home

- Your partner refuses to consider therapy or insists that you're the one who needs to change

Case Example 3: David's Difficult Decision David spent three years trying to make his relationship with Emma work despite her severe paranoid personality disorder. Emma was convinced that David was having multiple affairs, despite his complete faithfulness and transparency about his activities. She had installed spy software on all his devices, followed him to work, and contacted his colleagues to "investigate" his behavior.

David loved Emma and could see that she was suffering from her constant suspicions and anxiety. He tried everything—couple's therapy (which Emma used as an opportunity to present her "evidence" of his affairs), complete transparency about his activities, and even agreeing to give up friendships that made Emma suspicious.

Nothing worked. Emma's suspicions continued to escalate, and she began involving her family members in monitoring David's behavior. She would call David's mother to check his stories about family visits and contacted his employer with concerns about his "suspicious" work activities.

The turning point came when Emma accused David's teenage daughter (from a previous marriage) of helping to cover up his affairs. Emma began interrogating the daughter and monitoring her communications with David. David realized that Emma's paranoid disorder was now affecting an innocent child and that no amount of accommodation on his part would resolve her suspicions.

David made the difficult decision to end the relationship. Emma interpreted his departure as confirmation of all her suspicions, which was painful for David but also helped him understand that her paranoid thoughts would never be resolved by his actions.

When Love Meets Immovable Reality

Paranoid personality disorder presents unique challenges because it strikes at the foundation of all relationships—trust. Unlike other personality disorders where love and patience can sometimes create positive changes, paranoid personality disorder involves fixed beliefs that resist change even in the face of contradictory evidence.

The hardest part for partners is often accepting that your love, faithfulness, and transparency cannot cure your partner's paranoid thoughts. These thoughts arise from internal psychological patterns rather than external relationship dynamics. While you can learn to manage the symptoms and create some stability, you cannot prove your trustworthiness to someone whose brain interprets proof as further evidence of deception.

The decision to stay or leave must be based on your ability to live with these limitations while protecting your own mental health and safety. Some partners find ways to create sustainable relationships by setting clear boundaries and refusing to enable paranoid behaviors. Others realize that the constant suspicion and surveillance are incompatible with their needs for trust and emotional intimacy.

Key Takeaways

- Paranoid personality disorder involves pervasive distrust that affects all aspects of relationships, not just occasional jealousy

- Partners live under constant surveillance and suspicion, where innocence cannot be proven and trust cannot be rebuilt through evidence

- The paranoid mindset involves hypervigilance, confirmation bias, and attribution errors that make logical arguments ineffective

- Practical strategies include maintaining consistency, setting boundaries, and refusing to enable surveillance behaviors

- Safety planning becomes crucial when paranoid thoughts escalate to threats or dangerous behaviors

- The decision to continue these relationships requires honest assessment of whether the paranoid patterns are improving or worsening over time

Chapter 5: Schizoid Personality Disorder
- Loving a Ghost

You reach across the breakfast table to touch your partner's hand, and they don't pull away—but they don't respond either. It's like touching a statue. They're physically present but emotionally unreachable, existing in a world that seems to have room for only one person. You've learned to interpret the smallest gestures as signs of affection because grand emotional displays simply don't exist in their vocabulary. Sometimes you wonder if you're in a relationship or just sharing space with someone who tolerates your presence.

The Intimacy Paradox

They Want You Close But Need You Far

Schizoid personality disorder creates one of the most confusing relationship dynamics you'll encounter. Your partner chose to be in a relationship with you, which suggests they want connection. They may even say they love you and mean it genuinely. But their behavior suggests someone who would prefer to live as a hermit, showing little interest in emotional intimacy, social activities, or the typical expressions of love that most people expect in relationships.

According to Psychology Today research, people with schizoid personality disorder experience what psychologists call the "intimacy paradox." They have the same basic human need for connection as everyone else, but they also have an equally strong need for emotional distance and autonomy. This creates an internal conflict that plays out in relationships through confusing mixed signals and behaviors that can leave partners feeling rejected and confused.

The paradox manifests in several ways:

41

Physical Presence, Emotional Absence: They'll be physically available but emotionally distant, like being in the same room with someone who's mentally checked out.

Selective Engagement: They might engage deeply with intellectual topics, hobbies, or work but show little interest in emotional conversations or relationship discussions.

Parallel Lives: They prefer to coexist rather than actively participate in shared experiences, like two people living separate lives under the same roof.

Affection Without Intimacy: They might show care through practical actions (making sure you're fed, helping with tasks) but struggle with emotional expressions or physical affection.

Understanding this paradox helps explain why traditional relationship advice often fails with schizoid partners. They're not playing hard to get or trying to punish you—they're managing their own complex internal needs for both connection and distance.

Decoding Emotional Unavailability vs. Lack of Love

One of the most painful aspects of loving someone with schizoid personality disorder is constantly wondering if their emotional distance means they don't love you or if they're simply incapable of expressing love in conventional ways. This distinction matters enormously for your emotional well-being and your decisions about the relationship.

Signs of Schizoid Emotional Unavailability (which may coexist with genuine love):

- They struggle to express emotions verbally but may show care through actions

- They seem uncomfortable with your emotional expressions but don't ask you to stop

- They maintain consistent behavior toward you even if it's emotionally limited

- They make practical efforts to maintain the relationship (paying bills, showing up, staying faithful)

- They may occasionally share deeper thoughts or feelings in very safe contexts

- They seem content with the relationship even if they don't express enthusiasm

Signs That May Indicate Lack of Love:

- They seem irritated or burdened by your presence

- They actively avoid spending time with you or make excuses to be elsewhere

- They show no interest in your well-being, thoughts, or experiences

- They seem happier or more animated when you're not around

- They make no effort to maintain the relationship or participate in shared responsibilities

- They explicitly express that they'd prefer to be alone

Case Example 1: Mark's Silent Love Language Susan married Mark after a two-year courtship where his quiet, thoughtful nature attracted her. Mark was intelligent, reliable, and seemed to enjoy her company, though he was never emotionally expressive. Susan assumed that marriage would bring them closer and that Mark would become more open over time.

Five years into their marriage, Susan felt increasingly lonely and questioned whether Mark actually loved her. He rarely said "I love you," showed little physical affection, and seemed uninterested in the emotional conversations that Susan craved. Mark would sit quietly while Susan shared her feelings, offering minimal responses that left her feeling unheard and disconnected.

However, Susan began to notice that Mark expressed care in subtle but consistent ways. He would automatically make her coffee every morning exactly the way she liked it. When Susan was stressed about work, Mark would quietly handle household tasks without being asked. If Susan mentioned being interested in something, Mark would research it thoroughly and present her with detailed information or relevant items.

When Susan's father was hospitalized, Mark took time off work without being asked, drove Susan to the hospital every day, and handled all the logistics while Susan focused on her father. Mark didn't offer emotional comfort in traditional ways, but his practical support was unwavering and perfectly attuned to Susan's needs.

Susan realized that Mark did love her, but he expressed it through consistent actions rather than words or emotional displays. This understanding didn't solve all their relationship challenges, but it helped Susan stop interpreting Mark's emotional distance as rejection and start appreciating his unique way of showing love.

Building Connection Without Overwhelming

Creating intimacy with a schizoid partner requires abandoning conventional approaches to relationship building and developing strategies that respect their need for emotional space while still meeting your own needs for connection. This means learning to build bridges instead of trying to eliminate the distance between you.

Respect Their Processing Style: Schizoid personalities often need time to process emotions and experiences internally before they can share them externally. Instead of expecting immediate responses to emotional conversations, give them time and space to think before following up.

Find Their Natural Interests: Most people with schizoid personality disorder have areas of genuine interest and engagement, often intellectual or creative pursuits. Learning about these interests can provide natural connection points.

Use Indirect Communication: Direct questions about feelings might shut down conversation, but sharing your own experiences or asking about practical matters might open doors to deeper sharing.

Create Low-Pressure Opportunities: Instead of planning emotionally intensive date nights, create side-by-side activities where connection can happen naturally without pressure.

Appreciate Small Gestures: Learn to recognize and appreciate the subtle ways your partner shows care, rather than waiting for dramatic romantic gestures that may never come.

Maintain Your Own Social Needs: Don't expect your schizoid partner to meet all your social and emotional needs. Maintain friendships and activities that provide the social stimulation your partner cannot provide.

Finding Fulfillment When Your Partner Lives Behind Glass

The metaphor of loving someone behind glass captures the experience many partners describe—you can see them, you know they're there, but there's always a barrier that prevents full emotional contact. Learning to find fulfillment in this type of relationship requires adjusting expectations while maintaining your own emotional health.

Redefine Intimacy: Traditional intimacy might involve lengthy emotional conversations, frequent physical affection, and enthusiastic participation in shared activities. With a schizoid partner, intimacy might look like comfortable silence, shared intellectual interests, or simply being peacefully present in the same space.

Value Consistency Over Intensity: Schizoid partners often provide remarkable consistency in their care and presence, even if it lacks emotional intensity. Learning to value this steadiness can provide a different but meaningful form of security.

Find Meaning in Small Moments: Brief eye contact during a shared joke, a hand on your shoulder when you're upset, or a thoughtful observation about something you mentioned weeks ago might be your partner's version of grand romantic gestures.

Create Parallel Intimacy: Instead of trying to merge your emotional lives completely, find ways to share experiences while respecting each other's different emotional needs and processing styles.

Case Example 2: Building Bridges with Jennifer Rachel's partner Jennifer had schizoid personality disorder, which made traditional relationship building nearly impossible. Jennifer would shut down during emotional conversations, showed little interest in typical couple activities, and seemed most comfortable when they were doing separate activities in the same room.

Rachel initially tried to create more intimacy by planning romantic dinners, suggesting couple's therapy, and trying to have deep conversations about their relationship. All of these approaches made Jennifer more withdrawn and uncomfortable, which left Rachel feeling rejected and frustrated.

Eventually, Rachel discovered that Jennifer was most open during practical activities that didn't focus directly on emotions or relationships. When they worked together on home improvement projects, Jennifer would occasionally share thoughts about her childhood or observations about their relationship. When they watched documentaries together, Jennifer would make comments that revealed her thoughts and feelings indirectly.

Rachel learned to create opportunities for these natural moments of connection rather than forcing emotional conversations. She would share her own thoughts and feelings while doing dishes or during car rides, without expecting immediate responses from Jennifer. Over time, Jennifer began responding to these shares in her own quiet way.

Rachel also developed realistic expectations for their relationship. Instead of expecting passionate declarations of love, she appreciated Jennifer's consistent presence and the small ways Jennifer showed care. Instead of expecting enthusiasm for social activities, Rachel enjoyed Jennifer's companionship during quiet activities they both enjoyed.

Creating a Life That Works for Both of You

Successfully partnering with someone who has schizoid personality disorder requires creating a relationship structure that meets both people's needs without trying to change anyone's fundamental nature. This often means developing a more independent relationship style than many couples prefer.

Separate Together: Many successful couples with schizoid dynamics create homes and routines that allow for both connection and independence. This might mean separate offices or hobby spaces, parallel evening routines, or agreements about alone time.

Complementary Social Lives: The non-schizoid partner might maintain more active social relationships while the schizoid partner participates minimally or not at all. This requires agreements about social obligations and expectations.

Different Love Languages: Learn to appreciate and reciprocate your partner's unique ways of showing affection rather than expecting them to adapt to more conventional expressions of love.

Realistic Expectations: Accept that some typical relationship experiences (passionate romance, frequent emotional support, enthusiastic participation in social activities) may not be available, while other benefits (consistency, loyalty, peaceful companionship) may be stronger than in more emotionally intense relationships.

Personal Growth: Use the independence in your relationship as an opportunity for personal growth, pursuing interests and relationships that fulfill needs your partner cannot meet.

Case Example 3: Tom and Maria's Parallel Success Tom and Maria created a marriage that worked for both of them by accepting their different emotional needs and building a relationship that accommodated both. Maria had schizoid personality disorder and preferred minimal social interaction and emotional distance. Tom was more emotionally expressive and socially active.

Instead of trying to make Maria more social or Tom more independent, they created a life that honored both their needs. Tom maintained close friendships and participated in social activities, sometimes alone and sometimes with Maria's minimal participation. Maria had her own creative pursuits and quiet spaces in their home where she could retreat when she needed solitude.

They developed routines that provided connection without overwhelming Maria's need for space. They would have coffee together each morning, sharing practical information about their days but not requiring deep emotional conversation. They would spend evenings in the same room, Tom reading or socializing online while Maria worked on her art projects.

When Tom needed emotional support, he had learned to be direct about his needs rather than expecting Maria to intuit them. Maria had learned to offer practical support during Tom's difficult times, even if she couldn't provide emotional comfort in conventional ways.

Their relationship worked because both partners accepted their differences as personality variations rather than problems to be solved. Tom found fulfillment in his friendships and independent activities, while also appreciating Maria's steady presence and unique perspective. Maria felt secure in a relationship that didn't demand more emotional engagement than she could comfortably provide.

The Art of Loving Someone Who Lives Internally

Schizoid personality disorder challenges conventional ideas about what love looks like in relationships. Your partner may love you deeply while showing little emotional expression. They may be completely faithful and committed while seeming uninterested in typical romantic activities. They may provide remarkable consistency and practical support while struggling to offer emotional comfort.

Learning to love someone with schizoid personality disorder means learning a different language of love—one that's spoken through actions rather than words, through presence rather than passion, through consistency rather than intensity. It requires developing the ability to find connection in quiet moments and to appreciate forms of intimacy that don't match cultural expectations.

The key question isn't whether your partner loves you in conventional ways, but whether the way they do love you feels meaningful and sustainable for your own emotional needs. Some partners find deep satisfaction in these quieter forms of love. Others realize they need more emotional engagement than a schizoid partner can provide. Both responses are valid and deserve respect.

Key Takeaways

- Schizoid personality disorder creates an intimacy paradox where partners want connection but need emotional distance

- Emotional unavailability doesn't necessarily indicate lack of love—schizoid partners often show care through consistent actions rather than emotional expressions

- Building connection requires respecting their need for space while creating low-pressure opportunities for natural sharing

- Successful relationships often involve parallel lives with separate social needs and complementary relationship roles

- Redefining intimacy and adjusting expectations can help partners find fulfillment without trying to change their schizoid partner's fundamental nature

- The decision to continue these relationships depends on whether the available forms of love and connection meet your own emotional needs

Chapter 6: Schizotypal Personality Disorder

When Reality Isn't Shared

Your partner mentions casually that they think the new neighbor is sending them messages through the way he arranges his garden gnomes. They're completely serious. When you gently suggest that might not be the case, they look at you with a mixture of pity and frustration, clearly believing you're either naive or deliberately refusing to see what's obvious to them. These moments force you to navigate the delicate space between supporting someone you love and maintaining your own grip on reality.

Magical Thinking in Relationships

When Logic Fails

Schizotypal personality disorder brings a unique set of challenges to relationships because it affects how your partner perceives and interprets reality. Unlike other personality disorders that primarily impact emotional regulation or interpersonal behavior, schizotypal personality disorder involves differences in thought patterns, perception, and social cognition that can make your partner seem like they're living in a different world.

Magical thinking—the belief that thoughts, wishes, or rituals can influence events in ways that defy logical cause-and-effect relationships—is a hallmark of schizotypal personality disorder. Your partner might believe that:

- Coincidences have special meaning or represent signs from the universe

- They have special abilities to sense things others cannot

- Certain rituals or behaviors can influence outcomes in supernatural ways

- Random events are connected in meaningful patterns

- They can influence other people's thoughts or behavior through mental focus

- Objects, places, or people have special significance beyond their obvious properties

These beliefs aren't temporary phases or conscious choices—they represent genuine differences in how your partner's brain processes information and makes connections between events. Understanding this helps explain why logical arguments typically fail to change these beliefs and why your partner might seem confused or frustrated by your inability to see what seems obvious to them.

Case Example 1: Jennifer's Daily Navigation Jennifer had been dating Marcus for eight months when she realized that his quirky observations and insights weren't just creative thinking—they represented a fundamentally different way of experiencing reality. Marcus would make connections between seemingly unrelated events, convinced that patterns existed that others couldn't see.

For example, Marcus believed that the number of red cars he saw on his drive to work predicted how his day would go. He would adjust his route and timing based on these observations, sometimes arriving late to important meetings because the "signs" suggested he should wait. Marcus also thought that certain combinations of his clothing could influence other people's moods and behavior, spending significant time each morning choosing outfits based on the interactions he wanted to create that day.

Initially, Jennifer found Marcus's unique perspective interesting and even charming. But over time, she realized that his magical thinking affected practical aspects of their relationship. Marcus would interpret Jennifer's normal mood variations as responses to his thoughts about her. If he woke up worried about their relationship, he would assume Jennifer was picking up on his concerns telepathically and would spend the day trying to read hidden meanings in her ordinary responses.

When Jennifer tried to discuss these patterns logically, Marcus would become frustrated and accuse her of being closed-minded or unable to perceive the subtle connections he could see. This left Jennifer feeling confused about how to supportively engage with Marcus's beliefs without enabling thinking patterns that sometimes interfered with his work and social relationships.

Social Isolation and the Burden on Partners

People with schizotypal personality disorder often feel like outsiders in social situations, sensing that others find them odd or difficult to understand. Their unusual thought patterns, eccentric behaviors, and difficulty reading social cues can lead to gradual isolation from mainstream social connections. This isolation often places enormous pressure on romantic partners to meet all their social and emotional needs.

Your partner might:

- Avoid social gatherings because they feel uncomfortable or misunderstood

- Make observations or comments that others find strange or inappropriate

- Misinterpret social interactions, reading hostile intentions into neutral behaviors

- Feel more comfortable with you than with anyone else, leading to social overdependence

- Struggle to maintain friendships or professional relationships

- Prefer unusual or fringe social groups that accept their eccentric thinking

As the partner, you might find yourself becoming their primary social connection and interpreter of the outside world. This can feel flattering initially—your partner sees you as their safe person, their anchor to social reality. But over time, this role can become exhausting and isolating for you as well.

You might start avoiding social situations because you're never sure what your partner will say or how others will react. You might find yourself constantly translating between your partner's unique perspective and social expectations. You might feel responsible for managing your partner's social relationships and protecting them from rejection or misunderstanding.

Communication Strategies for the "Lost in Translation" Relationship

Communicating effectively with a schizotypal partner requires developing strategies that bridge the gap between your different ways of processing information and understanding social interactions. Traditional communication advice often fails because it assumes both partners share similar frameworks for interpreting events and relationships.

Validate Without Agreeing: You can acknowledge your partner's experiences without confirming their interpretations. For example: "I can see that this feels very meaningful to you" rather than "You're right that the universe is sending you signs."

Ask Curious Questions: Instead of challenging their beliefs directly, ask questions that might help them examine their thinking. "What makes you think that connection exists?" or "Have you noticed times when that pattern didn't hold true?"

Focus on Impact Rather Than Truth: When magical thinking creates practical problems, focus on the consequences rather than the validity of the beliefs. "I notice you've been late to work several times this week because of your driving route decisions. How do you think that's affecting your job?"

Establish Reality Anchors: Agree on certain facts or sources of information that you both trust, and refer back to these when discussions become too disconnected from shared reality.

Use Their Language: Learn to communicate in ways that respect their thinking patterns while still conveying important information. If they respond to symbolic thinking, use metaphors and analogies rather than purely logical arguments.

Case Example 2: Managing Daily Communication Challenges David learned to navigate communication with his girlfriend Sarah, who had schizotypal personality disorder, by developing strategies that worked with her thinking patterns rather than against them. Sarah would often interpret ordinary events as having special significance for their relationship, which would lead to confusion and conflict when David didn't share her interpretations.

For instance, Sarah believed that the appearance of certain animals during their walks together indicated the health of their relationship. If they saw couples (two birds, two squirrels), Sarah interpreted this as a positive sign. If they saw solitary animals, she would become worried about their future together. David initially tried to explain that animal behavior had nothing to do with their relationship, which led to arguments about his lack of spiritual awareness.

Eventually, David learned to acknowledge Sarah's observations without reinforcing the magical thinking. He would say things like "You notice a lot of details during our walks" or "It's interesting how you find meaning in the things around us." This validated Sarah's experience without confirming her interpretations.

55

When Sarah's magical thinking created practical problems—like wanting to reschedule important plans because she hadn't seen the "right" signs—David would focus on the consequences rather than challenging her beliefs directly. He would explain his own needs and limitations rather than arguing about the validity of her concerns.

David also learned to communicate his own feelings and needs clearly, because Sarah often misinterpreted his emotions or assumed she knew what he was thinking through intuitive means. He would be explicit about his mood, his plans, and his feelings rather than expecting Sarah to read social cues accurately.

Managing Family Events and Social Situations

One of the most challenging aspects of being partnered with someone who has schizotypal personality disorder involves managing social situations where their unusual thinking or behavior might create awkwardness or misunderstanding. This requires balancing your loyalty to your partner with your need to maintain other important relationships.

Preparation Strategies:

- Brief your partner on social expectations for specific events

- Discuss potentially challenging topics or situations beforehand

- Establish signals or phrases you can use if conversations become too unusual

- Plan ahead for how long you'll stay and when you might need to leave

- Prepare explanations for your partner's behavior that are honest but protective

During Social Events:

- Stay close enough to provide support but avoid hovering or appearing protective

- Redirect conversations gently when your partner's comments become too eccentric or concerning

- Have backup topics ready that engage your partner's interests in socially appropriate ways

- Monitor your partner's stress levels and suggest breaks or departures when needed

- Support your partner without enabling behavior that makes others genuinely uncomfortable

After Social Events:

- Debrief with your partner about what went well and what was challenging

- Address any social mistakes or misunderstandings with compassion rather than criticism

- Help your partner understand social reactions without making them feel rejected or abnormal

- Process your own feelings about the social dynamics with appropriate support people

Case Example 3: Jennifer's Family Navigation Jennifer faced ongoing challenges attending family gatherings with her boyfriend Alex, who had schizotypal personality disorder. Alex would make observations about family members that he believed were insightful but that others found intrusive or strange. He might comment on someone's "aura" or suggest that family conflicts were related to planetary alignments.

Jennifer's family liked Alex personally but found his comments unsettling and didn't know how to respond. Jennifer felt caught between protecting Alex from rejection and maintaining peace with her family. She also worried that Alex's behavior might affect her own relationships with family members.

Jennifer developed several strategies that helped manage these situations. Before family events, she would discuss the social context with Alex, explaining who would be there and what topics might be sensitive. She would remind Alex that not everyone shared his spiritual beliefs and suggest ways he could engage with family members around their interests rather than his metaphysical observations.

During gatherings, Jennifer would stay aware of conversations and gently redirect when Alex's comments were making others uncomfortable. She might say something like "Alex has such an interesting perspective on things" and then shift the conversation to more neutral topics. She also learned to recognize when Alex was becoming overwhelmed by social stimulation and would suggest breaks or early departures.

After events, Jennifer would acknowledge what went well while also helping Alex understand when his comments had confused or concerned others. She would explain social reactions in educational rather than critical ways, helping Alex learn to read social cues more effectively.

Most importantly, Jennifer had honest conversations with her family about Alex's personality differences, helping them understand that his unusual comments came from genuine belief systems rather than attempts to be difficult or attention-seeking. This context helped her family respond with more patience and curiosity rather than judgment or discomfort.

Professional Help

When and How to Suggest It Gently

People with schizotypal personality disorder often don't recognize that their thinking patterns differ significantly from others, which can make them resistant to suggestions about therapy or professional help. They might view their unique perceptions as gifts rather than symptoms, or they might fear that mental health professionals will try to eliminate aspects of their personality that they value.

However, professional help can be extremely beneficial for schizotypal personality disorder, particularly therapy approaches that focus on improving social skills, reality testing, and coping strategies rather than trying to eliminate all unusual thinking patterns.

Signs That Professional Help Might Be Beneficial:

- Your partner's magical thinking is interfering with work, relationships, or daily functioning

- They're experiencing distress about feeling different or misunderstood

- Social isolation is increasing and affecting their mental health

- Unusual perceptions or beliefs are becoming more intense or frequent

- They're struggling with anxiety or depression related to their social difficulties

- You're feeling overwhelmed by being their only source of social connection and reality checking

Approaches for Suggesting Professional Help:

Focus on Specific Goals: Rather than suggesting they need therapy for their personality, focus on specific areas where they've expressed frustration or where problems are occurring. "You mentioned feeling stressed about work relationships. There are therapists who specialize in helping people with social skills in professional settings."

Emphasize Enhancement Rather Than Change: Frame therapy as a way to enhance their natural abilities rather than fix problems. "A therapist could help you learn to communicate your insights in ways that others can understand better."

Suggest Couple's Therapy: Sometimes suggesting couple's therapy feels less threatening than individual therapy and can help address communication patterns while providing professional perspective.

Research Compatible Therapists: Look for mental health professionals who have experience with schizotypal personality disorder and who take approaches that respect individual differences rather than trying to impose conventional thinking patterns.

Be Patient with Resistance: Don't push too hard if your partner initially resists. Continue to model healthy communication and coping strategies while leaving the door open for future conversations about professional support.

Understanding the Limits of Your Influence

One of the most difficult aspects of loving someone with schizotypal personality disorder is accepting that you cannot serve as their primary reality check or social interpreter without significant cost to your own mental health. While your support and understanding are valuable, your partner's unusual thinking patterns and social difficulties require more comprehensive help than any single relationship can provide.

Your role as a partner involves:

- Providing emotional support and acceptance

- Learning communication strategies that work with their thinking patterns

- Helping them navigate social situations when appropriate

- Encouraging professional help when needed

- Maintaining your own mental health and social connections

Your role does not include:

- Serving as their only social connection

- Constantly correcting their perceptions or beliefs

- Managing all their social relationships for them

- Sacrificing your own social needs to accommodate their isolation

- Taking responsibility for their success in work or other relationships

Creating Boundaries That Protect Both of You

Healthy boundaries in schizotypal relationships require careful balance between supporting your partner's unique perspective and maintaining your own connection to social reality. These boundaries protect both your mental health and your partner's opportunity to develop their own coping skills.

Reality Testing Boundaries: Agree on limits regarding how much time you'll spend discussing or analyzing your partner's unusual beliefs or perceptions. While some discussion can be supportive, endless analysis can pull you into thought patterns that affect your own reality testing.

Social Responsibility Boundaries: Clarify what social situations you'll attend together and what level of support you can provide without feeling overwhelmed or embarrassed. Be honest about your own social needs and limitations.

Decision-Making Boundaries: Determine which decisions you'll make together using conventional logic and which decisions you'll allow your partner to make based on their own belief systems, even if you disagree.

Communication Boundaries: Establish limits on conversations that become too disconnected from shared reality, while still respecting your partner's need to share their experiences.

Professional Help Boundaries: Clarify that while you can provide emotional support, you cannot serve as your partner's therapist, social skills coach, or primary reality check.

Finding Peace in Different Worlds

Schizotypal personality disorder presents unique challenges because it affects the fundamental ways your partner perceives and interprets reality. Unlike other personality disorders where the primary issues involve emotional regulation or relationship patterns, schizotypal disorder requires partners to navigate differences in basic cognition and worldview.

The key to sustainable relationships with schizotypal partners often involves learning to appreciate their unique perspectives while maintaining your own grounding in consensual reality. This means finding ways to honor their different way of experiencing the world without losing yourself in their belief systems or becoming their sole anchor to conventional social expectations.

Success in these relationships doesn't require your partner to abandon all their unusual thinking patterns or for you to accept all their beliefs as valid. Instead, it requires developing mutual respect for different ways of processing information and creating agreements about how to navigate practical life together despite these differences.

Some partners find deep meaning and growth in these relationships, appreciating their partner's creative and spiritual insights while helping them develop better social skills. Others realize that the cognitive and social differences create too much stress or isolation for sustainable partnership. Both outcomes reflect honest assessment of compatibility rather than failure or success.

Key Takeaways

- Schizotypal personality disorder involves differences in thought patterns and reality perception, not just emotional or social difficulties

- Magical thinking represents genuine beliefs about how the world works, not conscious choices or attempts to be difficult

- Communication strategies must bridge different frameworks for interpreting events and relationships

- Social isolation often places excessive pressure on romantic partners to meet all social and emotional needs

- Professional help can be beneficial but requires gentle, goal-focused approaches that respect individual differences

- Healthy boundaries protect both partners while allowing space for unique perspectives and conventional reality testing

Chapter 7: Antisocial Personality Disorder

The Dangerous Dance

The charming stranger who sweeps you off your feet during the first three months of dating slowly reveals a different face. What seemed like confidence becomes ruthless manipulation. What felt like passion becomes calculated control. The person who promised you the world begins systematically dismantling your world—your finances, your relationships, your sense of reality. You find yourself trapped in a relationship with someone who views other people as objects to be used rather than human beings deserving of respect and care.

Red Flags You Wished You'd Seen Sooner

Antisocial personality disorder creates some of the most dangerous relationship dynamics you'll encounter. Unlike other personality disorders that stem from emotional dysregulation or attachment difficulties, antisocial personality disorder involves a fundamental lack of empathy and conscience. People with this condition don't experience guilt, remorse, or genuine concern for others' wellbeing in the way most people do.

The early warning signs often get overlooked because they're masked by intense charm and attention. People with antisocial personality disorder can be incredibly charismatic in the beginning, making you feel like the most important person in their world. This isn't genuine love—it's a calculated strategy to gain your trust and access to what you can provide.

Early Red Flags Include:

Excessive Charm and Flattery: They come on strong, declaring love quickly and making grand promises about your future together. This feels amazing initially but represents love-bombing—a manipulation tactic designed to make you emotionally dependent.

Inconsistent Life Stories: Details about their past change depending on their audience. They might tell you different versions of the same events, or their stories about work, family, or previous relationships don't add up when you pay close attention.

Financial Irregularities: They might have unexplained wealth, constantly changing jobs, legal troubles they dismiss as misunderstandings, or they quickly become interested in your financial situation.

Relationship to Rules and Authority: They consistently break small rules and social norms, always having excuses for bad behavior. They view themselves as exceptions to normal standards and become angry when held accountable.

Treatment of Service Workers: Watch how they treat waiters, cashiers, or anyone in service positions. People with antisocial personality disorder often show contempt for people they perceive as beneath them or unable to benefit them.

Lack of Long-term Relationships: They may not have close friendships or family relationships, or they'll have dramatic stories about how previous partners "betrayed" them or "couldn't handle" their success.

Case Example 1: The Perfect Beginning Gone Wrong Rachel met Marcus at a professional conference where he was presenting on innovative business strategies. Marcus was articulate, well-dressed, and seemed successful and confident. He approached Rachel after her own presentation, complimenting her work and suggesting they continue their conversation over dinner.

During their early dates, Marcus was incredibly attentive. He would send flowers to Rachel's office, plan elaborate dates, and talk about their future together after just a few weeks of dating. He seemed fascinated by Rachel's work in nonprofit management and her connections in the community. Marcus shared stories about his own successful consulting business and his plans to expand internationally.

The first red flag appeared when Rachel invited Marcus to a work function. She introduced him to colleagues, and later discovered he had given different people completely different explanations of his business and background. When Rachel asked him about the inconsistencies, Marcus became defensive and accused her colleagues of misunderstanding his work.

Over the following months, more concerning patterns emerged. Marcus would disappear for days without explanation, then return with elaborate stories about business emergencies or family crises. He began borrowing small amounts of money, always with promises to repay quickly, but never following through. When Rachel expressed concern about these patterns, Marcus would alternate between intense apologies and anger, accusing Rachel of not trusting him or supporting his success.

By the time Rachel realized she was dealing with someone who manipulated others for personal gain, Marcus had borrowed thousands of dollars, had access to her professional network, and had isolated her from friends who had expressed concerns about his behavior.

Manipulation vs Mental Illness

One of the most challenging aspects of antisocial personality disorder relationships is distinguishing between behavior caused by mental illness and behavior that represents calculated manipulation. This distinction matters enormously for your safety and decision-making.

Most personality disorders involve people who struggle with their symptoms and experience distress about their relationship difficulties. People with borderline personality disorder feel genuine anguish about their relationship instability. People with avoidant personality disorder suffer from their social fears. Their behaviors, while challenging, stem from internal pain and genuine attempts to manage overwhelming emotions.

Antisocial personality disorder operates differently. The behaviors that harm others don't cause the person with antisocial personality disorder to experience distress. They don't feel guilty about lying, manipulating, or exploiting others. They don't experience remorse about the pain they cause. This isn't because they're evil—it's because their brain doesn't process empathy and conscience the way most people's brains do.

Mental Illness Characteristics (found in other personality disorders):

- The person experiences distress about their symptoms

- They show genuine remorse when they hurt others

- They want to change problematic behaviors

- Their harmful behaviors stem from emotional dysregulation or fear

- They can form some genuine emotional connections with others

Manipulative/Antisocial Characteristics:

- The person doesn't experience distress about harming others

- They show no genuine remorse—any apologies are strategic rather than heartfelt

- They only want to change behaviors that cause consequences for them personally

- Their harmful behaviors are calculated to achieve specific goals

- Their emotional connections to others are shallow and self-serving

Understanding this distinction helps explain why the relationship strategies that work with other personality disorders often fail catastrophically with antisocial personality disorder. Empathy, understanding, and patience—valuable tools in most relationship challenges—become vulnerabilities that antisocial personalities exploit.

Creating Your Exit Strategy

If you're in a relationship with someone who has antisocial personality disorder, your safety must be your primary concern. Unlike other personality disorders where the relationship might be salvageable with appropriate boundaries and professional help, antisocial personality disorder relationships typically become more dangerous over time as the person becomes more comfortable showing their true nature.

Creating an exit strategy isn't about giving up on love—it's about protecting yourself from someone who views you as an object to be used rather than a person to be cherished.

Immediate Safety Planning:

1. **Secure Your Finances**: Change passwords on all financial accounts. If you share accounts, start moving money to accounts they cannot access. Document any money they've taken or promised to repay.

2. **Protect Your Identity**: Secure important documents like passport, birth certificate, social security card. Check your

credit reports for any accounts or charges you didn't authorize.

3. **Document Everything**: Keep records of concerning behaviors, threats, financial exploitation, or other problematic incidents. Take photos of any destroyed property or evidence of their deception.

4. **Maintain Outside Relationships**: Don't let them isolate you from friends and family. These relationships will be crucial for emotional support and practical help during your exit.

5. **Create Safe Communication**: Have ways to communicate that they cannot monitor—separate phone, email account, or communication apps they don't know about.

6. **Plan Your Physical Safety**: Have places you can go immediately if you feel unsafe. Keep some essentials (clothes, medications, important documents) in an easily accessible location.

Case Example 2: Lisa's Calculated Escape Lisa recognized the signs of antisocial personality disorder in her boyfriend Jake after two years of increasingly disturbing behavior. Jake had systematically isolated Lisa from her friends by creating conflicts with them, had gained access to her business accounts through manipulation, and had become increasingly controlling and threatening when Lisa questioned his behavior.

Lisa realized that a direct confrontation with Jake would be dangerous. People with antisocial personality disorder often become vengeful when they lose control over their victims. Instead, Lisa developed a careful exit strategy that protected her safety and assets.

First, Lisa secured her finances by opening new accounts at a different bank and gradually moving her money. She changed all her passwords and set up alerts for any unusual account activity. She discovered that Jake had been using her credit cards without permission and had opened accounts in her name, so she worked with a financial advisor to clean up her credit and protect her assets.

Lisa reconnected with friends Jake had driven away, explaining the situation and asking for support. She was surprised to discover that several friends had been concerned about Jake's behavior but hadn't known how to express their worries without seeming judgmental.

Lisa documented Jake's threatening behaviors and financial exploitation, keeping records in a safe location outside their shared home. She consulted with both a therapist experienced in abusive relationships and a lawyer about the best way to safely end the relationship and protect herself legally.

When Lisa finally told Jake the relationship was over, she did so with friends present and with a plan to stay elsewhere immediately. As predicted, Jake became enraged and threatening, alternating between promises to change and threats about what would happen if Lisa left him. Having prepared for this reaction, Lisa was able to stay safe while Jake exhausted his manipulation tactics.

Legal Considerations and Protecting Your Assets

Relationships with antisocial personalities often involve financial exploitation, identity theft, property destruction, or other illegal activities. Protecting yourself legally requires understanding both your rights and the likely tactics your partner might use during and after the relationship ends.

Financial Protection Strategies:

Credit Monitoring: Set up alerts with all three credit bureaus to monitor for new accounts, inquiries, or changes to your credit report. People with antisocial personality disorder often use partners' identities to obtain credit or make purchases.

Account Security: Change all passwords and security questions for financial accounts. Remove your partner's access to any shared accounts or credit cards. If you have joint accounts, work with your bank to understand your options for protecting your assets.

Document Financial Abuse: Keep records of any money they've taken, promised to repay, or used without permission. Take photos of receipts, bank statements, or other evidence of financial exploitation.

Legal Documentation: If your partner has stolen money, used your identity, or destroyed your property, document these crimes. You may need this evidence for restraining orders, criminal charges, or civil proceedings.

Property Protection: If you live together, understand your legal rights regarding shared property. Document valuable items that belong to you, and have important possessions moved to safe locations if possible.

Professional Legal Advice: Consult with an attorney who has experience with domestic abuse cases. They can help you understand your rights and options for protecting yourself legally and financially.

Case Example 3: Tom's Legal Nightmare and Recovery Tom discovered that his girlfriend Sarah had been systematically stealing from him for months. Sarah had access to Tom's home office where he kept financial documents for his small business. She had been making copies of checks, using his business credit card for personal purchases, and had even filed fraudulent tax returns using his business information.

When Tom confronted Sarah about these activities, she initially denied everything, then claimed she had borrowed the money intending to repay it, and finally became threatening about what she would do if Tom involved authorities. Sarah told Tom she would claim he had been abusive and would ruin his business reputation if he pursued legal action.

Tom realized he was dealing with someone who had no conscience about stealing or making false accusations. He immediately consulted with both a criminal attorney and a family law attorney to understand his options and protect himself.

Working with his attorneys, Tom documented all the financial crimes, secured his business accounts and assets, and filed appropriate reports with law enforcement. He also obtained a restraining order that prevented Sarah from contacting him or coming to his workplace.

The legal process was lengthy and expensive, but Tom eventually recovered most of his stolen money and prevented Sarah from causing further damage to his business. More importantly, he learned to recognize the signs of antisocial behavior and developed better boundaries to protect himself from future exploitation.

Healing from Psychological Warfare

Recovery from an antisocial personality disorder relationship involves more than just ending the relationship and recovering financially. These relationships often involve psychological abuse that affects your ability to trust your own perceptions, make good decisions, and form healthy relationships in the future.

Common Psychological Effects:

Reality Distortion: Constant lies and manipulation can make you question your own memory and perceptions. You may find yourself second-guessing your instincts or feeling confused about what really happened in various situations.

Emotional Numbness: The constant stress of dealing with manipulation and exploitation can lead to emotional shutdown as a protective mechanism. You might feel disconnected from your own emotions or unable to experience joy and excitement.

Hypervigilance: After being constantly deceived and manipulated, you may become overly suspicious of others' motives, even in safe relationships. This protective mechanism can interfere with your ability to form new connections.

Self-Blame and Shame: You may feel embarrassed about "falling for" the manipulation or blame yourself for not seeing the signs sooner. These feelings can prevent you from seeking help or forming new relationships.

Trust Issues: After being betrayed by someone you loved, you may struggle to trust anyone, including friends, family members, and potential romantic partners who are genuinely trustworthy.

Recovery Strategies:

Professional Support: Work with a therapist who has experience with psychological abuse and manipulation. They can help you process your experiences and develop healthy coping strategies.

Reality Anchoring: Reconnect with trusted friends and family members who can help you remember your worth and validate your experiences. These relationships provide perspective and emotional support.

Self-Compassion: Practice treating yourself with the same kindness you would offer a friend in your situation. You were targeted by someone skilled at manipulation—this doesn't reflect any failure or weakness on your part.

Gradual Trust Building: Start rebuilding your ability to trust by engaging with people in low-risk situations. Notice how trustworthy people behave differently from those with antisocial traits.

Education and Awareness: Learn about antisocial personality disorder and manipulation tactics. Understanding these patterns helps prevent future victimization and reduces self-blame about past experiences.

Bottom Line Truths

Antisocial personality disorder represents one of the most dangerous relationship dynamics because it involves someone who fundamentally lacks empathy and conscience. Unlike other personality disorders where love and patience might create positive change, antisocial personality disorder typically worsens over time as the person becomes more comfortable showing their true nature.

The most important message for anyone dealing with this situation is that your safety matters more than trying to save or change someone who views you as an object rather than a person. These relationships don't improve with understanding, compassion, or accommodation—they improve only when you remove yourself from harm's way.

Recovery from these relationships is possible, but it requires accepting the reality of what you experienced and taking active steps to protect and heal yourself. You deserve relationships based on mutual respect, genuine care, and emotional safety. Recognizing antisocial patterns early and prioritizing your wellbeing aren't acts of selfishness—they're acts of wisdom and self-preservation.

Key Insights for Partners

- Antisocial personality disorder involves calculated manipulation rather than emotional dysregulation, making traditional relationship strategies dangerous and ineffective

- Early red flags include excessive charm, inconsistent stories, financial irregularities, and lack of genuine empathy for others

- Safety planning must prioritize physical and financial protection, as these relationships often escalate in danger over time

- Legal protection involves securing assets, documenting abuse, and working with attorneys experienced in domestic abuse cases

- Recovery requires professional support to address psychological effects like reality distortion, hypervigilance, and trust issues

- Unlike other personality disorders, antisocial relationships rarely improve with time, patience, or understanding

Chapter 8: Borderline Personality Disorder

Riding the Emotional Rollercoaster

The morning starts with your partner telling you they've never been happier, that you're the love of their life, that everything feels perfect between you. By evening, they're accusing you of planning to leave them, threatening to hurt themselves if you don't prove your commitment, and listing every way you've disappointed them over the past month. This isn't just a bad day—it's Tuesday. And Wednesday will likely bring yet another dramatic swing between desperate love and furious abandonment fears.

The Push-Pull Cycle

Why They Fear Losing You But Push You Away

Borderline personality disorder creates one of the most confusing relationship dynamics you'll encounter because it involves contradictory impulses happening simultaneously. Your partner desperately fears abandonment while engaging in behaviors that push you away. They crave intimacy while feeling terrified of vulnerability. They want you close but feel suffocated by closeness. This isn't manipulative game-playing—it's the result of a brain that struggles to regulate emotions and maintain stable relationships.

According to Psych Central research, people with borderline personality disorder experience emotions with an intensity that most people can't imagine. What might feel like mild frustration to you registers as rage in their nervous system. What seems like a minor disagreement triggers their deepest abandonment fears. Their emotional reactions aren't proportional to situations because their brain's threat-detection system is hypersensitive and their emotional regulation skills are underdeveloped.

The push-pull cycle typically follows predictable patterns:

The Pull Phase (I need you desperately):

- Intense declarations of love and commitment

- Wanting to spend all available time together

- Making grand plans for your shared future

- Extreme anxiety when you're apart or unavailable

- Interpreting your independence as signs of rejection

The Push Phase (I hate you/You're going to leave me anyway):

- Sudden anger or criticism about perceived slights

- Testing behaviors designed to see if you'll abandon them

- Threats to end the relationship before you can leave them first

- Self-destructive behaviors that create relationship crises

- Interpreting your efforts to help as proof that something is wrong

This cycle exhausts both partners. You never know which version of your partner you'll encounter from day to day or even hour to hour. Just when you think you've found stability, the cycle repeats.

Case Example 1: David's Emotional Whiplash David met Amanda during a particularly stable period in her life. Amanda had just started a new job she enjoyed, had been consistently attending therapy, and seemed to have her borderline personality disorder symptoms well-managed. Their early relationship felt intense but positive—Amanda was passionate about their connection and made David feel like the most important person in her world.

Six months into their relationship, Amanda's job became stressful due to a difficult manager. This external stress triggered Amanda's borderline symptoms, and David found himself caught in cycles he didn't understand. On Monday, Amanda would be planning their vacation together and talking about moving in together. By Thursday, she would be accusing David of being emotionally unavailable and threatening to break up because he "obviously" didn't care about her as much as she cared about him.

The accusations confused David because they seemed to come from nowhere. He would cancel plans with friends to spend more time with Amanda, only to have her accuse him of being suffocating. He would give her space when she seemed overwhelmed, only to have her interpret his distance as rejection and abandonment.

David started walking on eggshells, constantly trying to read Amanda's emotional state and adjust his behavior accordingly. He began avoiding topics that might upset her and stopped sharing his own concerns because Amanda would interpret his problems as signs that he was pulling away from their relationship.

The relationship became a constant crisis management situation where David felt responsible for Amanda's emotional stability but had no reliable way to predict or prevent her emotional storms.

DBT Skills Every Partner Needs to Know

Dialectical Behavior Therapy (DBT) was specifically designed to help people with borderline personality disorder learn emotional regulation skills. According to Cleveland Clinic research, DBT teaches four core skill sets that can benefit not only the person with borderline personality disorder but also their partners who are trying to navigate these challenging relationship dynamics.

Understanding these skills helps you respond more effectively to borderline behaviors and protect your own mental health during emotional crises.

Distress Tolerance Skills:

These skills help you cope with crisis situations without making them worse. During your partner's emotional storms, your natural instinct might be to fix the problem, argue about facts, or become emotional yourself. Distress tolerance skills help you stay grounded and avoid escalating the situation.

- **STOP Technique**: Stop what you're doing, Take a breath, Observe the situation objectively, Proceed with intention rather than reaction

- **Distract**: Use activities to shift focus away from the crisis until emotions decrease to manageable levels

- **Self-Soothe**: Use your five senses to comfort yourself (calming music, warm bath, favorite scent, soft textures, comforting tastes)

- **Improve the Moment**: Use imagery, meaning-making, prayer/meditation, or relaxation to make crisis moments more tolerable

Emotional Regulation Skills:

These skills help you manage your own emotional responses to your partner's instability while also modeling healthy emotional management.

- **PLEASE**: Treat Physical illness, balance Eating, avoid mood-Altering substances, balance Sleep, get Exercise

- **Opposite Action**: Act opposite to your emotional impulse when your emotions don't fit the facts (approach instead of avoid when anxious, be gentle instead of angry when frustrated)

- **Emotional Labeling**: Identify and name emotions specifically rather than getting overwhelmed by intensity

Interpersonal Effectiveness Skills:

These skills help you maintain your own needs and boundaries while staying connected to your partner during difficult times.

- **DEAR MAN**: Describe the situation, Express your feelings, Assert your needs, Reinforce positive outcomes, stay Mindful, Appear confident, Negotiate when possible

- **GIVE**: be Gentle in approach, act Interested, Validate their experience, use Easy manner

- **FAST**: be Fair, avoid Apologies when not warranted, Stick to values, be Truthful

Mindfulness Skills:

These skills help you stay present and avoid getting pulled into the emotional chaos while maintaining awareness of your own needs and limits.

- **Observe**: Notice thoughts, feelings, and sensations without immediately reacting

- **Describe**: Put experiences into words without judgment or interpretation

- **Participate**: Fully engage in the present moment rather than getting lost in worry about the future or regret about the past

Case Example 2: Learning to Surf Instead of Drowning Maria learned to use DBT skills to navigate her relationship with her boyfriend Carlos, who had borderline personality disorder. Before learning these skills, Maria would get pulled into Carlos's emotional crises, spending hours trying to talk him through his fears and anger, which usually made situations worse rather than better.

Maria learned to use the STOP technique when Carlos became escalated. Instead of immediately trying to fix his emotional state, she would pause, breathe, and observe what was actually happening versus what Carlos's emotions were telling him was happening. This helped her avoid getting swept into his emotional experience.

When Carlos would accuse Maria of not loving him enough (usually triggered by something minor like Maria mentioning plans with friends), Maria learned to validate his feelings without accepting false accusations. She would say things like "I can see you're really scared right now" instead of defending herself against unfair criticisms or trying to prove her love through grand gestures.

Maria used distress tolerance skills during Carlos's self-harm threats or relationship ultimatums. Instead of panic-managing the crisis, she would stay calm, ensure immediate safety, and avoid making promises or decisions based on crisis emotions. This approach actually helped Carlos learn to manage his own emotions better because he couldn't rely on Maria's emotional reactions to regulate his feelings.

Most importantly, Maria learned to maintain her own needs and boundaries even during Carlos's emotional storms. She would offer support within her limits but wouldn't sacrifice her own well-being to manage his emotional state.

Managing Crisis Without Losing Yourself

One of the biggest challenges in borderline relationships is maintaining your own identity and emotional stability while dealing with frequent crises. According to HelpGuide.org research, partners often develop secondary trauma from constant emotional chaos, losing their ability to recognize their own needs and maintain healthy boundaries.

Crisis Management Strategies:

Safety First: During threats of self-harm or suicide, your primary responsibility is ensuring immediate safety, not managing your partner's emotions. Call crisis hotlines, involve mental health professionals, or call emergency services when necessary. Don't try to handle serious safety threats alone.

Stay Grounded in Reality: Borderline emotions are intense but often temporary. Avoid making major decisions or commitments based on crisis emotions. Keep perspective about what's actually happening versus what emotions are making the situation feel like.

Limit Crisis Conversations: Set boundaries about how long you'll spend discussing the same crisis or concerns. Endless analysis often increases emotional intensity rather than providing resolution.

Maintain Your Schedule: Don't consistently cancel your own plans or activities to manage your partner's crises. This teaches both of you that their emotional state controls your life, which increases rather than decreases their abandonment fears.

Use Support Systems: Have people you can call for perspective and emotional support. Don't try to handle borderline relationship challenges alone.

Document Patterns: Keep track of triggers, cycles, and what approaches help versus harm. This information can be valuable for treatment and helps you maintain perspective during intense moments.

Setting Boundaries with Someone Who Has No Boundaries

People with borderline personality disorder often struggle with appropriate boundaries due to their intense fear of abandonment and difficulty regulating emotions. They might read your texts, show up unannounced, demand constant reassurance, or involve others in your relationship conflicts. Setting boundaries feels mean or rejecting to you, but clear limits actually create the safety and predictability that help reduce borderline symptoms.

Boundary Setting Framework:

Be Clear and Specific: Vague boundaries don't work with borderline personalities. Instead of "I need space," say "I need two hours without phone calls to finish this work project, then I'll call you back."

Start Small: Begin with boundaries you can consistently maintain rather than trying to fix everything at once. Success with small boundaries builds skills for larger ones.

Expect Testing: Your partner will likely push against new boundaries to see if you'll maintain them. This isn't necessarily manipulative—it's often anxiety about whether you'll abandon them if they make mistakes.

Stay Calm During Pushback: Maintain boundaries without becoming angry or defensive. Emotional reactions often escalate borderline behaviors rather than reducing them.

Follow Through Consistently: Inconsistent boundaries create more anxiety than no boundaries because they create unpredictability about what to expect.

Case Example 3: Boundaries That Actually Worked Sarah learned to set effective boundaries with her girlfriend Jessica, who had borderline personality disorder, after months of feeling like she had no privacy or personal space. Jessica would read Sarah's text messages, demand detailed explanations about Sarah's activities, and become hysterical if Sarah didn't respond to calls immediately.

Sarah's first boundary was about phone communication during work. She explained to Jessica that she couldn't answer personal calls during work hours but would call back during lunch and after work. Initially, Jessica panicked about this limit, interpreting it as rejection and lack of love.

Sarah stayed consistent with the boundary despite Jessica's emotional reactions. She would send a brief text saying "At work, will call at lunch as promised" but wouldn't engage in lengthy text conversations or take crisis calls unless there were genuine emergencies.

Within two weeks, Jessica began to adapt to this routine and actually felt more secure knowing when to expect contact from Sarah. The predictability reduced her abandonment anxiety better than constant contact had.

Sarah gradually added other boundaries—Jessica couldn't read her texts, couldn't make unplanned visits to Sarah's workplace, and couldn't involve Sarah's family in their relationship conflicts. Each boundary required patience and consistency, but over time they created a more stable relationship dynamic.

Most importantly, Sarah maintained these boundaries with compassion rather than anger. She would explain that the limits weren't about loving Jessica less but about creating a relationship structure that worked for both of them.

When Love is Enough vs When It's Time to Go

The most difficult question in borderline relationships is distinguishing between a challenging but workable relationship and one that's become harmful to your mental health. Love alone isn't enough to sustain these relationships, but love combined with the right skills, professional support, and genuine effort from both partners can create stable, satisfying connections.

Signs the Relationship May Be Workable:

Your Partner Seeks Help: They're engaged in therapy, taking prescribed medications, and genuinely trying to learn better coping skills rather than expecting you to manage their emotional state.

Abuse is Absent: While borderline behaviors can be intense and dramatic, the relationship doesn't involve physical violence, threats, financial exploitation, or other forms of abuse.

You Can Maintain Your Identity: You're able to keep your own friends, interests, and goals rather than having your entire life consumed by managing your partner's emotional needs.

Crises Decrease Over Time: While emotional intensity might remain high, actual crises (self-harm, threats, relationship ultimatums) become less frequent as your partner develops better coping skills.

Communication is Possible: During calm periods, you can discuss relationship issues and your partner can acknowledge their role in problems rather than blaming everything on external circumstances.

Signs It May Be Time to Leave:

Your Mental Health is Deteriorating: You're developing anxiety, depression, or trauma symptoms from the constant emotional chaos and crisis management.

Abuse is Present: Any form of physical violence, threats, financial exploitation, or systematic attempts to control your behavior indicates a dangerous situation.

No Professional Help: Your partner refuses therapy, won't take prescribed medications, or expects you to be their sole source of emotional support and crisis management.

Increasing Isolation: You've lost important relationships, career opportunities, or personal goals due to the demands of managing your partner's emotional state.

No Improvement Over Time: Despite your efforts and possibly professional help, the relationship patterns are staying the same or getting worse rather than gradually improving.

The decision to stay or leave should be based on realistic assessment of whether the relationship is moving toward greater stability and mutual respect or remaining stuck in destructive patterns that harm both partners.

The Reality of Loving Someone with Borderline Patterns

Borderline personality disorder relationships can work when both partners understand the condition, develop appropriate skills, and have access to professional support. These relationships often involve more emotional intensity than many people prefer, but they can also include deep connection, passion, and growth when managed skillfully.

The key is recognizing that your love and support, while valuable, cannot cure borderline personality disorder. Professional treatment is typically necessary for significant improvement. Your role involves learning to respond effectively to borderline behaviors while maintaining your own mental health and boundaries.

Success in these relationships requires accepting that emotional intensity may always be higher than in other relationships while working toward reducing harmful behaviors and increasing emotional stability. Both partners must be willing to learn new skills and make changes to create a sustainable dynamic.

Key Insights for Partners

- The push-pull cycle stems from simultaneous fears of abandonment and intimacy, creating contradictory behaviors that aren't intentionally manipulative

- DBT skills help both partners manage emotional intensity and develop healthier communication patterns during crises

- Crisis management requires prioritizing immediate safety while avoiding decisions based on temporary emotional states

- Boundaries with borderline partners must be specific, consistent, and maintained with compassion rather than anger

- Professional treatment is typically necessary for significant improvement—love and support alone aren't sufficient

- The decision to continue these relationships should be based on whether patterns are improving and both partners can maintain their mental health and personal growth

Chapter 9: Histrionic Personality Disorder

The Spotlight Stealer

You're at dinner with friends, sharing exciting news about a promotion at work, when your partner suddenly develops a mysterious illness that requires immediate attention. Or you're comforting a friend through a difficult time when your partner arrives with dramatic news about their own crisis that somehow seems more urgent than anyone else's problems. You begin to notice a pattern—every gathering, every conversation, every moment that doesn't center on your partner somehow gets redirected back to them through theatrical displays of emotion, sudden emergencies, or captivating stories that demand everyone's focus.

Life as a Supporting Actor in Your Own Relationship

Histrionic personality disorder transforms relationships into ongoing theatrical productions where your partner always plays the starring role and everyone else serves as supporting cast. This isn't conscious selfishness or deliberate attention-seeking—people with histrionic personality disorder genuinely feel uncomfortable and anxious when they're not the center of attention. Their brain interprets being ignored or overlooked as a form of rejection that triggers intense emotional distress.

Your partner with histrionic personality disorder experiences the world as their personal stage. They need constant validation, admiration, and emotional responses from others to feel secure and worthwhile. When attention shifts away from them, even briefly, they may unconsciously create situations that redirect focus back to their needs, emotions, or experiences.

This creates an exhausting dynamic where you find yourself constantly in a supporting role, even in situations that should be about you. Your achievements get overshadowed by their reactions to your achievements. Your problems get minimized in favor of their more dramatic concerns. Your social gatherings become performances where your partner entertains while you manage the logistics and smooth over any social disruptions their dramatic behavior might create.

Common Spotlight-Stealing Behaviors:

Emotional Escalation: When others are receiving attention, your partner might suddenly become very upset, excited, or dramatic about something unrelated, forcing everyone to shift focus to their emotional state.

Crisis Creation: Mysterious illnesses, sudden emergencies, or urgent problems that coincidentally appear when attention is directed elsewhere.

Story Competition: Every story someone tells triggers a bigger, more dramatic, or more interesting story from your partner that captivates the audience.

Physical Dramatics: Exaggerated gestures, theatrical expressions, costume-like clothing choices, or attention-grabbing behaviors that ensure they remain visually prominent.

Emotional Intensity: Expressing emotions with such intensity that others feel compelled to respond, comfort, or engage with their feelings rather than continuing previous conversations.

Case Example 1: Maria's Exhausting Performance Schedule David noticed the pattern six months into his relationship with Maria. Every time they attended social gatherings, Maria would somehow become the center of attention through dramatic stories, emotional displays, or sudden needs that required everyone's concern. At first, David found Maria's vivacious personality attractive—she was never boring, always had interesting stories, and seemed to light up every room she entered.

But David began to feel invisible in his own life. When David received recognition at work, Maria would suddenly have a crisis with her boss that required hours of emotional support and analysis. When David's father was hospitalized, Maria developed mysterious symptoms that demanded medical attention during the same week, making it difficult for David to focus on his family emergency.

At social gatherings, David watched friends initially engage with Maria's entertaining stories and emotional expressions, but over time, people began to seem exhausted by her constant need for reactions and validation. David found himself apologizing for Maria's dramatic behaviors or trying to redirect conversations to include other people, which often triggered more intense attention-seeking from Maria.

David realized he had become Maria's stage manager rather than her partner. His role involved setting up situations where Maria could shine, managing the social fallout from her dramatic behaviors, and sacrificing his own social and emotional needs to keep Maria's spotlight burning brightly.

Attention-Seeking vs Narcissism

Histrionic personality disorder is often confused with narcissistic personality disorder because both conditions involve behaviors that seem self-centered and attention-seeking. However, the underlying motivations and emotional experiences are quite different, which affects how you approach the relationship and what strategies might be helpful.

Histrionic Attention-Seeking Characteristics:

- Stems from anxiety and insecurity rather than grandiosity

- The person genuinely enjoys other people and wants to connect, even if their methods are problematic

- They can feel empathy for others but may struggle to express it appropriately

- They want to be liked and admired by everyone, not just to be seen as superior

- Their dramatic behaviors often feel childlike or innocent rather than calculating

- They can sometimes recognize their attention-seeking patterns and feel embarrassed about them

Narcissistic Attention-Seeking Characteristics:

- Stems from feelings of superiority and entitlement to special treatment

- The person views others as sources of admiration rather than genuine connection

- They struggle with empathy and may not care about others' feelings unless it affects them

- They want to be seen as better than others, not just liked by others

- Their attention-seeking often involves putting others down or highlighting their superiority

- They rarely recognize problematic patterns and become defensive when confronted

Understanding this distinction helps you respond more effectively. Histrionic behaviors often respond to gentle redirection, validation of their underlying insecurity, and consistent but kind boundaries. Narcissistic behaviors typically require firmer boundaries and less emotional engagement because empathy and understanding get interpreted as weakness rather than love.

Case Example 2: The Difference in Daily Life Jennifer's relationship with Mark (histrionic patterns) felt very different from her previous relationship with Alex (narcissistic patterns), even though both partners seemed to need constant attention and admiration.

Mark would create dramatic situations and tell elaborate stories, but his goal seemed to be entertaining others and getting positive reactions. When Jennifer's friends expressed annoyance with Mark's attention-seeking, he would feel genuinely hurt and embarrassed, often apologizing and trying to modify his behavior. Mark wanted everyone to like him and was distressed when his dramatic behaviors created social problems.

In contrast, Alex had viewed other people as an audience for his superiority rather than individuals he wanted to connect with. Alex would monopolize conversations by talking about his achievements and would become angry rather than embarrassed when people seemed tired of his self-promotion. Alex wanted to be admired but didn't particularly care if people actually liked him as a person.

Mark's attention-seeking had an anxious, insecure quality—he seemed genuinely afraid that people would lose interest in him if he wasn't constantly entertaining. Alex's attention-seeking had an entitled, demanding quality—he seemed to believe that others owed him admiration and became resentful when it wasn't provided automatically.

This difference affected how Jennifer could respond to each partner. With Mark, gentle conversations about social balance and reassurance about her affection could sometimes reduce his attention-seeking behaviors. With Alex, these approaches were interpreted as Jennifer being too demanding or not appreciating his specialness.

Practical Strategies for the Exhausted Partner

Living with histrionic personality disorder requires specific strategies that acknowledge your partner's genuine need for attention and validation while protecting your own energy and ensuring that your needs also get met within the relationship. Traditional relationship advice about compromise and understanding often falls short because it doesn't account for the intensity and consistency of histrionic attention needs.

Managing Daily Attention Needs:

Scheduled Spotlight Time: Designate specific times when your partner has your full attention for sharing stories, discussing their feelings, or simply being the focus of conversation. This predictable attention can reduce their anxiety about being overlooked.

Positive Attention for Appropriate Behavior: Notice and respond when your partner shows interest in others, asks questions about your experiences, or shares attention appropriately in social situations.

Redirect Rather Than Ignore: When your partner interrupts or redirects conversations inappropriately, gently guide them back to appropriate social engagement rather than ignoring their attempts at connection.

Validate Underlying Feelings: Acknowledge their need for connection and validation while addressing problematic behaviors. "I can see you want to be part of this conversation" followed by guidance about appropriate ways to engage.

Social Situation Management:

Prepare in Advance: Before social gatherings, discuss expectations and agreements about sharing attention, letting others talk, and showing interest in other people's experiences.

Use Signals: Develop subtle ways to communicate when your partner's attention-seeking is becoming problematic, allowing them to modify their behavior without public embarrassment.

Practice Turn-Taking: Help your partner learn to ask questions about others and wait for responses rather than immediately redirecting conversations back to themselves.

Plan Recovery Time: Social situations that require attention-sharing can be exhausting for histrionic personalities. Plan quiet time afterward where they can have your full attention.

Finding Your Voice in a One-Person Show

One of the most challenging aspects of histrionic relationships is maintaining your own identity and voice when your partner's personality naturally dominates social situations and relationship dynamics. You might find yourself becoming quieter, more background-focused, or losing confidence in your own experiences and opinions because they seem less dramatic or interesting than your partner's constant stream of stories and emotions.

Strategies for Maintaining Your Voice:

Claim Your Own Story Time: Don't wait for natural openings in conversations—histrionic personalities may not create them. Instead, deliberately claim time and space for your own experiences and thoughts.

Set Communication Boundaries: Establish limits on how long your partner can monopolize conversations or require attention before you also get to share or before the conversation includes other topics.

Maintain Independent Relationships: Have friendships and social connections where your partner isn't present and you can be the primary speaker and center of attention when appropriate.

Practice Self-Advocacy: Learn to interrupt appropriately when your partner redirects conversations away from your experiences. "I wasn't finished sharing about my day" or "Let me finish this thought first."

Develop Your Own Interests: Pursue activities, hobbies, and goals that are entirely yours and don't require your partner's participation or approval. This helps maintain your sense of individual identity.

Case Example 3: Sarah Finds Her Stage Sarah realized she had become nearly invisible in her relationship with Tommy, who had histrionic personality disorder. Tommy wasn't malicious—he genuinely loved Sarah and wanted to share his life with her. But his constant need for attention and dramatic storytelling meant that Sarah rarely got to share her own experiences or thoughts without them being overshadowed by Tommy's more theatrical responses.

Sarah started small by claiming specific times for her own sharing. During their evening check-ins, Sarah would say, "I need ten minutes to tell you about my day before we discuss yours." Initially, Tommy would interrupt with related stories or emotional reactions, but Sarah learned to say, "Let me finish first, then I want to hear your response."

Sarah also began maintaining friendships separately from Tommy. She joined a book club where Tommy wasn't present, allowing her to express her own opinions and have conversations where she wasn't competing with dramatic storytelling for attention.

Most importantly, Sarah learned to appreciate her own quieter, more reflective communication style instead of feeling inadequate compared to Tommy's theatrical expressions. She realized that not everything needed to be dramatic to be meaningful, and that her thoughtful observations and steady support were valuable even if they didn't command immediate attention.

Creating Space for Your Own Needs

Histrionic relationships often become so focused on managing your partner's emotional needs and attention requirements that your own needs get forgotten or minimized. This isn't usually intentional—your partner may genuinely care about your wellbeing but struggle to notice your needs when they're not expressed as dramatically as their own.

Need Identification and Expression:

Be Explicit About Your Needs: Don't expect your histrionic partner to notice subtle signs that you need support, attention, or care. Express your needs directly and specifically rather than hoping they'll be intuited.

Schedule Your Own Crisis Time: If your partner gets immediate attention during emotional crises, establish that you also deserve focused attention when you're struggling, even if your distress is less dramatic.

Maintain Non-Negotiable Self-Care: Protect time and activities that restore your energy and maintain your mental health, regardless of your partner's attention needs or emotional state.

Create Emotional Space: Don't feel obligated to match your partner's emotional intensity or to have dramatic reactions to their dramatic presentations. You can be supportive while maintaining your own emotional equilibrium.

Seek Outside Validation: Make sure you have relationships and activities that provide validation and attention for your own experiences, achievements, and perspectives.

The Art of Loving a Performer

Histrionic personality disorder relationships can be rewarding when you learn to appreciate your partner's genuine warmth and enthusiasm while maintaining your own identity and needs. These partners often bring excitement, creativity, and emotional richness to relationships that can be deeply fulfilling when balanced appropriately.

The key lies in understanding that your partner's need for attention stems from insecurity rather than selfishness, which means it can often be managed through reassurance, boundaries, and skill-building rather than criticism or withdrawal. Unlike narcissistic personalities who view attention as their due, histrionic personalities typically respond well to gentle guidance about appropriate social behavior and mutual attention-sharing.

Success requires learning to direct your partner's dramatic tendencies in positive ways while ensuring that your own voice and needs remain visible in the relationship. This might mean teaching them to channel their storytelling abilities into entertaining others appropriately, or helping them learn to show interest in other people's experiences as a way of connecting rather than competing.

Key Insights for Partners

- Histrionic personality disorder involves genuine anxiety about being overlooked rather than entitled demands for special treatment

- Attention-seeking behaviors stem from insecurity and can often be reduced through reassurance and appropriate boundary-setting

- Partners must actively maintain their own voice and identity to avoid becoming supporting actors in someone else's performance

- Practical strategies include scheduled attention time, social preparation, and explicit communication about needs and boundaries

- Success requires appreciating your partner's warmth and enthusiasm while ensuring mutual attention-sharing and respect for both partners' experiences

- These relationships can be fulfilling when dramatic tendencies are channeled positively and both partners' needs are acknowledged and met

Chapter 10: Narcissistic Personality Disorder

Surviving the Hall of Mirrors

The relationship begins like a fairy tale. You've never felt so special, so understood, so cherished. Your new partner seems to see qualities in you that you didn't even know you possessed, showering you with attention that feels intoxicating after years of more ordinary relationships. But somewhere along the way, the fairy tale transforms into something much darker. The person who once elevated you to goddess status now seems to find fault with everything you do. The admiration in their eyes has been replaced by criticism, contempt, and a coldness that makes you question everything you thought you knew about love and about yourself.

The Idealize-Devalue-Discard Cycle Explained

According to Charlie Health research, narcissistic personality disorder relationships follow a predictable pattern that leaves partners feeling confused and psychologically battered. This cycle isn't random or based on your behavior—it's a systematic process that reflects how narcissistic personalities manage their internal sense of inadequacy and their need to maintain psychological control over others.

The Idealization Phase (You're Perfect): During this phase, you experience what feels like the most intense love of your life. Your partner seems captivated by everything about you, makes grand romantic gestures, and treats you like you're the most amazing person they've ever encountered. This isn't genuine love—it's a projection. They're not seeing the real you; they're seeing an idealized version that makes them feel special by association.

The idealization serves several functions for the narcissistic personality. It makes you emotionally dependent on their approval and attention. It establishes them as someone with exceptional taste and judgment (after all, they "discovered" your specialness). And it creates a baseline of treatment that they can later withdraw as a form of control and punishment.

The Devaluation Phase (You're Disappointing): Once you're emotionally invested and your life has become intertwined with theirs, the criticism begins. Nothing you do is quite right anymore. The qualities they once praised become sources of irritation. Your independence becomes "selfishness." Your kindness becomes "weakness." Your success becomes threatening to their sense of superiority.

This phase is designed to break down your self-esteem and make you work harder to regain their approval. The criticism is often subtle at first—small comments about your appearance, your choices, or your character that gradually erode your confidence. Over time, the devaluation becomes more obvious and more devastating.

The Discard Phase (You're Worthless): Eventually, when you're no longer serving their psychological needs or when they've found a new source of admiration, narcissistic personalities will discard you with shocking coldness. The person who once claimed you were their soulmate will treat you like you never mattered at all. They may disappear without explanation, replace you quickly with someone else, or become openly hostile and cruel.

The discard is designed to leave you questioning your own worth and reality. Many people spend years trying to understand what they did wrong or how they could regain the love they experienced during idealization, not realizing that the "love" was never real—it was a manipulation tactic.

Case Example 1: Tom's Three-Year Nightmare Tom met Elena at a professional conference where she was a keynote speaker. Elena seemed impressed by Tom's intelligence and career achievements, and their initial conversations were exciting and intellectually stimulating. Elena pursued Tom actively, calling him brilliant, telling him she'd never met someone who understood her work so well, and making plans for them to attend conferences together as a power couple.

The first six months felt like the relationship Tom had always dreamed of. Elena would introduce him to her professional network as her "brilliant partner," would seek his advice on her presentations, and would make him feel like an equal participant in her successful career. Tom began restructuring his own work schedule to accommodate Elena's travel and to be available when she needed intellectual support.

The shift began subtly. Elena started making small comments about Tom's presentation style, suggesting that he wasn't as polished as her other professional contacts. She would correct his grammar in public, dismiss his ideas as "interesting but not quite right," and began introducing him as "my boyfriend" rather than highlighting his professional accomplishments.

By the second year, Elena's criticism had become constant and devastating. She would analyze Tom's social interactions and point out everything he did wrong. She would compare him unfavorably to her ex-partners and professional colleagues. She would withdraw affection and attention whenever Tom didn't meet her changing and impossible standards.

The discard happened suddenly when Elena met another professional who impressed her. Elena became cold and distant, eventually telling Tom that she had realized they weren't compatible and that she needed someone more ambitious and sophisticated. Elena moved on to her new relationship immediately, leaving Tom devastated and questioning everything he thought he knew about himself and about love.

Gaslighting

Recognizing When Reality is Being Rewritten

Gaslighting represents one of the most psychologically damaging aspects of narcissistic abuse. According to research from Choosing Therapy and Talkspace, gaslighting involves systematically making you question your own perceptions, memories, and sanity through deliberate manipulation of information and emotional reactions.

Narcissistic personalities use gaslighting to maintain control and to avoid accountability for their behavior. Instead of acknowledging their mistakes or cruel treatment, they convince you that your perceptions are wrong, your memory is faulty, or your emotional reactions are unreasonable.

Common Gaslighting Tactics:

Denial of Events: "That never happened," "You're imagining things," or "You're being paranoid" when you confront them about their behavior.

Minimization: "You're overreacting," "It wasn't that bad," or "You're too sensitive" when you express hurt about their treatment.

Blame Shifting: "You made me do that," "If you hadn't provoked me," or "You're the one with the problem" when confronted about harmful behavior.

Rewriting History: Changing details of past events to make themselves look better or you look worse, often with such confidence that you begin to doubt your own memory.

Emotional Invalidation: "You're crazy," "You're too emotional," or "No one else would react this way" when you have normal emotional responses to their behavior.

Reality Distortion: Creating alternative explanations for events that sound plausible but shift responsibility away from them and onto you or external circumstances.

The goal of gaslighting is to make you dependent on the narcissistic person's version of reality because you can no longer trust your own perceptions. This creates psychological control that's more powerful than physical force because it attacks your ability to recognize and resist manipulation.

Case Example 2: Recognizing the Manipulation Lisa spent three years in a relationship with Marcus before she realized the extent to which he had been manipulating her perception of reality. Marcus would make cruel comments about Lisa's appearance, intelligence, or social skills, then deny saying them when Lisa brought up her hurt feelings.

Lisa began writing down incidents immediately after they happened because Marcus's denials were so convincing that she started questioning her own memory. When Lisa showed Marcus her notes, he accused her of being "obsessive" and "creating problems where none existed."

Marcus would also reinterpret Lisa's emotional reactions to make her seem irrational. When Lisa became upset about Marcus flirting with other women at parties, Marcus would say, "Your jealousy is really unattractive and it's pushing me away." When Lisa tried to discuss relationship problems, Marcus would say, "You're always creating drama—no wonder your previous relationships failed."

The most damaging aspect was Marcus's ability to make Lisa feel like she was the problem in their relationship. He would point out that all their conflicts started when Lisa brought up concerns, that she was the one who seemed unhappy, and that maybe she wasn't mature enough for a serious relationship.

Lisa finally recognized the gaslighting when a friend pointed out that Lisa had changed dramatically since dating Marcus. Lisa used to be confident and outgoing, but now she constantly second-guessed herself and seemed anxious about expressing any opinions or needs. This outside perspective helped Lisa realize that Marcus's version of reality didn't match anyone else's observations of their relationship.

Gray Rock and Other Survival Techniques

When you're dealing with narcissistic abuse—particularly when you can't immediately leave the relationship due to financial, legal, or family obligations—survival techniques can help protect your mental health and reduce the narcissistic person's ability to manipulate and control you.

Gray Rock Technique: This approach involves making yourself as uninteresting as possible to the narcissistic person. You become like a gray rock—present but boring, unresponsive to their attempts to provoke emotional reactions. This reduces their interest in targeting you because narcissistic personalities feed on emotional reactions and drama.

Gray rock involves:

- Giving brief, factual responses without emotional content

- Avoiding sharing personal information, feelings, or opinions

- Not reacting to insults, provocations, or attempts to start arguments

- Keeping conversations focused on necessary practical matters only

- Avoiding eye contact and emotional engagement during interactions

Information Diet: Limit what personal information you share with the narcissistic person. They often use your vulnerabilities, dreams, fears, and personal details as ammunition for future attacks or manipulation. Share only what's absolutely necessary for practical purposes.

Documentation: Keep records of abusive incidents, threats, financial manipulation, or other concerning behaviors. This serves multiple purposes—it helps you maintain perspective when they deny or minimize their behavior, it provides evidence if you need legal protection, and it helps you recognize patterns that might be difficult to see when you're in the middle of the situation.

Support Network Protection: Don't isolate yourself, even though the narcissistic person may pressure you to cut ties with friends and family. Maintain relationships with people who knew you before the narcissistic relationship and can provide reality checks and emotional support.

Financial Protection: If possible, maintain some financial independence and protect important documents. Narcissistic personalities often use financial control as a manipulation tool, so having your own resources provides options for escape if necessary.

Protecting Children from Narcissistic Dynamics

If you have children with a narcissistic partner, protecting them from psychological damage becomes a primary concern that affects all your decisions about the relationship. Children are particularly vulnerable to narcissistic manipulation because they naturally depend on parents for emotional security and reality testing.

How Narcissistic Parents Harm Children:

Golden Child/Scapegoat Dynamics: Narcissistic parents often designate one child as perfect (golden child) and another as the source of all problems (scapegoat), creating unhealthy competition and confusion among siblings.

Emotional Parentification: Children may be forced to manage the narcissistic parent's emotions, provide constant validation, or serve as confidants for adult problems they're not equipped to handle.

Reality Distortion: Children learn they can't trust their own perceptions because the narcissistic parent constantly rewrites reality to serve their own purposes.

Conditional Love: Children learn that love and acceptance depend on meeting the narcissistic parent's changing and impossible standards, creating lifelong struggles with self-worth.

Triangulation: Using children as messengers, allies, or weapons in conflicts with the other parent or other family members.

Protection Strategies:

Validate Children's Reality: When the narcissistic parent gaslights or manipulates children, provide gentle reality checks. "I saw what happened, and your feelings make sense."

Teach Emotional Skills: Help children identify and express their emotions in healthy ways, since narcissistic parents often invalidate or manipulate children's feelings.

Maintain Consistency: Be the stable, predictable parent who provides security and unconditional love, countering the narcissistic parent's unpredictable approval.

Avoid Competing: Don't try to be the "better" parent or put children in the middle of adult conflicts. Focus on being healthy and supportive rather than winning their loyalty.

Professional Help: Consider therapy for children who are showing signs of anxiety, depression, or behavioral problems related to the narcissistic parent's treatment.

Document Everything: Keep records of concerning incidents involving the children, as this information may be necessary for custody decisions or legal protection.

The Recovery Roadmap for Partners

Recovery from narcissistic abuse is a process that takes time and often requires professional support. The psychological damage from gaslighting, emotional abuse, and systematic devaluation affects your ability to trust yourself, form healthy relationships, and maintain appropriate boundaries with others.

Immediate Recovery Needs:

Reality Restoration: Work on trusting your own perceptions and memories again. Journal writing, therapy, and conversations with trusted friends can help you reconstruct accurate understanding of what happened in the relationship.

Emotional Regulation: Learn to identify and express your own emotions after years of having them invalidated or manipulated. You may have become disconnected from your feelings as a survival mechanism.

Self-Worth Rebuilding: Counter the narcissistic person's systematic attacks on your value and character by reconnecting with your authentic strengths, accomplishments, and positive qualities.

Boundary Development: Learn to recognize and maintain healthy boundaries in relationships, since narcissistic abuse often involves systematic boundary violations that leave you confused about what's acceptable treatment.

Long-term Recovery Goals:

Trauma Processing: Work through the psychological trauma of emotional abuse, which can create symptoms similar to PTSD including hypervigilance, emotional numbing, and difficulty trusting others.

Relationship Skills: Learn to recognize healthy relationship patterns and red flags for narcissistic or other abusive personalities in future relationships.

Identity Reconstruction: Reconnect with your authentic self, interests, and goals after years of having your identity shaped by someone else's needs and criticisms.

Trust Restoration: Gradually rebuild your ability to trust others while maintaining appropriate caution and boundary-setting skills.

Case Example 3: Sarah's Two-Year Recovery Journey Sarah left her marriage to David after five years of increasing narcissistic abuse, but she quickly realized that ending the relationship was only the beginning of her recovery process. Sarah had developed anxiety, depression, and a complete inability to trust her own judgment about people and situations.

Sarah started individual therapy with someone experienced in narcissistic abuse recovery. The therapist helped Sarah understand that her constant self-doubt and anxiety were normal responses to years of gaslighting and emotional manipulation rather than signs of mental illness or personal weakness.

Sarah also joined a support group for survivors of narcissistic abuse, where she met other people who had similar experiences. Hearing others describe the same manipulation tactics and psychological effects helped Sarah realize that David's treatment had been deliberately abusive rather than the result of relationship problems or her own inadequacies.

Recovery involved rebuilding Sarah's sense of reality by validating her experiences and memories of the abuse. Sarah learned to trust her instincts again by starting with small decisions and gradually working up to bigger life choices. She practiced setting boundaries with safe people before attempting to date again.

After two years of focused recovery work, Sarah was able to form a healthy relationship with someone who respected her boundaries, valued her opinions, and treated her with consistent kindness. The contrast helped Sarah fully understand how abnormal and damaging her marriage to David had been.

The Mirror Reveals Truth

Narcissistic personality disorder relationships represent some of the most psychologically damaging dynamics because they systematically attack your sense of reality, self-worth, and ability to trust your own perceptions. Unlike other personality disorders where the person struggles with their symptoms, narcissistic personalities typically don't experience distress about their behavior and rarely seek to change.

Recovery from these relationships requires understanding that the abuse was deliberate and systematic rather than the result of relationship problems or personal inadequacies. The "love" you experienced during idealization wasn't real—it was a manipulation tactic designed to create emotional dependence and control.

The most important message for survivors is that your experiences were real, your reactions were normal, and your worth isn't determined by how a narcissistic person chose to treat you. These relationships can teach you valuable lessons about boundaries, red flags, and your own strength, but they don't define your capacity for love or your value as a person.

Key Insights for Partners

- The idealize-devalue-discard cycle is a systematic manipulation pattern rather than normal relationship ups and downs

- Gaslighting attacks your ability to trust your own perceptions and represents one of the most damaging forms of psychological abuse

- Survival techniques like gray rock and information diet can protect your mental health when you can't immediately leave the relationship

- Children in narcissistic households need protection from psychological manipulation and reality distortion

- Recovery from narcissistic abuse takes time and often requires professional support to restore reality testing and self-worth

- These relationships teach valuable lessons about boundaries and red flags but don't reflect your actual worth or capacity for healthy love

Chapter 11: Avoidant Personality Disorder

Breaking Through the Walls

Your partner sits in the corner at every party, declining invitations to join conversations and seeming to shrink into themselves when people try to include them. They've turned down three promotions at work because they're terrified of the increased visibility and responsibility. They want desperately to connect with others but interpret every neutral expression as disapproval, every delayed text response as rejection. You find yourself becoming their social translator, their buffer against a world that feels perpetually hostile to them, while wondering how to love someone who seems to live in constant fear of your judgment too.

Fear of Rejection

When "No" Feels Like Abandonment

According to NCBI research, avoidant personality disorder represents one of the most painful personality disorders for both the person experiencing it and their loved ones. Unlike schizoid personality disorder where people genuinely prefer solitude, people with avoidant personality disorder desperately want close relationships but are paralyzed by their fear of rejection, criticism, and social humiliation.

The fear runs much deeper than normal social anxiety. Your partner's brain interprets neutral facial expressions as disapproval, delayed responses as rejection, and constructive feedback as devastating criticism. This hypersensitivity to potential rejection creates a self-fulfilling prophecy where they avoid social situations, relationships, and opportunities that could actually provide the connection and success they crave.

The NCBI studies show that people with avoidant personality disorder experience physical symptoms of anxiety in social situations—racing heart, sweating, nausea, and overwhelming urges to escape. But the emotional pain runs even deeper. They live with constant shame about their perceived inadequacies and overwhelming fear that others will discover how "defective" they believe themselves to be.

How Rejection Sensitivity Manifests in Relationships:

Catastrophic Interpretations: Your partner might interpret your tired expression after work as proof that you're losing interest in them, or your need for alone time as evidence that they're too boring or clingy.

Pre-emptive Withdrawal: Rather than risk rejection, they might reject first—pulling back emotionally or creating conflicts that give them a reason to retreat before you can abandon them.

Excessive Reassurance Seeking: They might need constant validation that you still love them, that they haven't done anything wrong, or that you're not planning to leave them.

Perfectionism Born of Fear: They might try to be the perfect partner, never expressing needs or disagreeing with you, because they believe any conflict will result in abandonment.

Social Isolation: They might avoid your friends and family, not because they don't want to connect, but because they're terrified of being judged and found wanting.

Case Example 1: Rachel's Journey Through Fear Rachel met James at the library where they both spent Saturday afternoons reading. James seemed thoughtful and intelligent, though incredibly shy. Their relationship developed slowly, with James seeming to need extensive reassurance before each step—holding hands, their first kiss, meeting Rachel's friends.

At first, Rachel found James's careful approach endearing. He seemed to treasure every moment they spent together and was incredibly attentive to her moods and needs. But gradually, Rachel realized that James's attentiveness came from anxiety rather than natural consideration. He was constantly monitoring her expressions, tone of voice, and body language for signs that she was becoming dissatisfied with him.

James would panic if Rachel seemed tired or distracted, immediately assuming he had done something wrong. He would ask repeatedly if she was upset with him, if she still wanted to be together, and what he could do to fix whatever he had done wrong. These conversations were exhausting for Rachel, who found herself constantly reassuring James about normal relationship dynamics.

The pattern became more pronounced when Rachel suggested James meet her family. James became physically ill at the thought, convinced that Rachel's parents would immediately see his flaws and convince Rachel to break up with him. James spent weeks preparing for the meeting, researching topics he thought Rachel's parents might find interesting and practicing conversations in front of the mirror.

Even after the successful meeting—Rachel's parents liked James and thought he was kind and intelligent—James remained convinced that they were just being polite and that they secretly thought Rachel could do better. This pattern of catastrophic thinking made it nearly impossible for James to enjoy positive experiences or believe in his own worth.

Building Safety in the Relationship Space

Creating emotional safety for someone with avoidant personality disorder requires understanding that their hypervigilance about rejection isn't paranoia—it's a deeply ingrained survival mechanism developed in response to early experiences of criticism, rejection, or emotional unavailability. Your role involves creating predictable, non-threatening interactions that gradually help your partner's nervous system learn that intimacy doesn't always lead to pain.

Establishing Predictable Safety:

Consistent Communication Patterns: Develop routines around how you check in with each other, express affection, and handle conflicts. Predictability reduces anxiety because your partner doesn't have to constantly guess what to expect from you.

Explicit Reassurance: While most people can infer love from actions, avoidant personalities often need verbal confirmation. Regular, explicit statements about your feelings help counter their constant fear that you're losing interest.

Gentle Conflict Resolution: Disagreements feel like catastrophic threats to someone with avoidant personality disorder. Learn to address issues using "I" statements, focusing on specific behaviors rather than character criticisms, and providing immediate reassurance that conflicts don't threaten the relationship.

Respect for Withdrawal Needs: When your partner becomes overwhelmed, give them space to retreat without making it about your relationship. "Take the time you need, and I'll be here when you're ready" provides safety without abandonment.

Celebrate Small Risks: When your partner tries something socially challenging—meeting new people, expressing a different opinion, or sharing a vulnerable feeling—acknowledge their courage rather than focusing on the outcome.

Helping Without Enabling Avoidance

The challenge in avoidant personality disorder relationships lies in providing support that encourages growth rather than enabling continued isolation. Your natural instinct might be to protect your partner from situations that cause them anxiety, but this protection often reinforces their avoidance patterns and prevents them from developing confidence through positive experiences.

Supporting Growth vs Enabling Avoidance:

Encouraging Gradual Exposure: Support your partner in taking small social risks rather than avoiding all challenging situations. This might mean attending a small gathering together rather than skipping all social events.

Processing Experiences Together: Help your partner examine their catastrophic predictions against actual outcomes. "You were worried that my coworkers would think you were boring, but did you notice how engaged they were when you talked about your photography?"

Avoiding Rescue Behaviors: Don't consistently speak for your partner in social situations or handle all interactions with service providers, authority figures, or new people. This prevents them from building their own social skills and confidence.

Validating Feelings While Challenging Thoughts: Acknowledge that social situations feel scary for your partner while gently questioning their worst-case scenario thinking. "I understand you're nervous about the dinner party, and it makes sense that meeting new people feels risky. What's the worst thing you think could realistically happen?"

Setting Limits on Reassurance: While some reassurance is necessary, endless reassurance-seeking can become a compulsion that increases rather than decreases anxiety. Set gentle limits: "I've told you three times that I love you and I'm happy with you. Let's practice believing that rather than asking again."

Case Example 2: Finding the Balance Between Support and Growth
Lisa learned to support her husband Mark's growth while avoiding the trap of becoming his social crutch. Mark had avoidant personality

disorder and would become physically ill before any social event, often finding excuses to cancel at the last minute or asking Lisa to make excuses for his absence.

Initially, Lisa would call their friends to explain that Mark wasn't feeling well or had work emergencies. She would attend events alone and field questions about why Mark never seemed to be able to join them. Lisa thought she was being supportive, but she realized she was actually enabling Mark's avoidance and making it easier for him to continue isolating.

Lisa started requiring that Mark make his own excuses when he chose to skip social events. This was terrifying for Mark initially, but it forced him to face the social consequences of his choices rather than hiding behind Lisa's explanations. Lisa discovered that when Mark had to explain his own absences, he became more motivated to attend events rather than face the awkward conversations about why he wasn't participating.

Lisa also stopped speaking for Mark in social situations. When friends asked Mark questions directly, Lisa would remain silent and let Mark respond, even if his answers were brief or awkward. This helped Mark develop his own voice and social skills rather than relying on Lisa to manage all interpersonal interactions.

Most importantly, Lisa learned to validate Mark's feelings while encouraging growth. Instead of saying "Don't worry, it will be fine" (which minimized his fears), Lisa would say "I know social situations feel scary for you, and I'm proud of you for being willing to try. What's one thing you could do to make this feel a little safer?"

Navigating Social Situations as a Couple

Social events present particular challenges for couples where one partner has avoidant personality disorder. Your partner wants to connect with others and be part of your social world, but they also feel overwhelmed by the potential for judgment and rejection. Successful social navigation requires planning, patience, and strategies that honor both your social needs and your partner's limitations.

Pre-Event Preparation:

Information Gathering: Help your partner feel less anxious by providing information about who will be there, what the setting will be like, and what types of conversations might occur. Unknown situations feel more threatening than predictable ones.

Escape Planning: Having an exit strategy reduces anxiety because your partner knows they're not trapped. Agree in advance on signals that indicate when your partner needs to leave and how you'll handle early departures gracefully.

Role Rehearsal: Practice conversations your partner might have, including responses to common questions about their work, interests, or opinions. This preparation builds confidence and reduces the fear of not knowing what to say.

Realistic Goal Setting: Instead of expecting your partner to be socially dynamic, set achievable goals like "stay for one hour," "have one conversation with someone new," or "ask one person about their interests."

During Events:

Stay Physically Close: Your presence provides security, so avoid leaving your partner alone with strangers for extended periods, especially early in the evening.

Include Without Spotlighting: Gently include your partner in conversations without putting them on the spot. "Mark was just telling me about his photography project" gives them a natural entry point without pressure to perform.

Monitor Stress Levels: Watch for signs that your partner is becoming overwhelmed—fidgeting, withdrawal, or very brief responses—and provide opportunities for breaks or quiet conversations.

Validate Efforts: Acknowledge your partner's courage in attending and participating, regardless of how successful they feel the interaction was.

Celebrating Small Victories

Progress with avoidant personality disorder happens in tiny increments that might be invisible to others but represent enormous courage for your partner. Learning to recognize and celebrate these small victories helps build momentum and reinforces your partner's growing confidence in their ability to handle social challenges.

Small Victories Worth Celebrating:

Initiating Social Contact: When your partner texts a friend, accepts a phone call, or suggests getting together with someone, acknowledge the effort this required.

Expressing Disagreement: If your partner shares a different opinion or expresses a preference that might cause conflict, celebrate their willingness to risk disapproval.

Trying New Activities: Whether it's ordering something different at a restaurant or joining a hobby group, new experiences require significant courage for avoidant personalities.

Recovering from Social Mistakes: When your partner bounces back from an awkward interaction or embarrassing moment, celebrate their resilience rather than focusing on what went wrong.

Asking for Help: Requesting assistance feels like admitting inadequacy to someone with avoidant personality disorder, so celebrate these moments of vulnerability.

Case Example 3: Tom's Gradual Progress Sarah learned to recognize and celebrate the incremental progress her boyfriend Tom made as he worked on his avoidant personality disorder. Tom's progress was often so subtle that Sarah initially missed the significance of his small steps forward.

Tom's first major victory was calling to make his own dental appointment rather than asking Sarah to do it for him. This seemed like a minor task to Sarah, but for Tom, it represented overcoming his fear of judgment from the receptionist and his anxiety about scheduling conflicts or not having the right information available.

Sarah started keeping a mental note of Tom's small victories—the day he disagreed with her about which movie to see, the evening he called his brother instead of avoiding the phone call, the morning he wore a colorful shirt instead of his usual neutral colors that helped him blend into the background.

Most significantly, Tom joined a photography club after months of wanting to but being too scared to attend meetings. Sarah celebrated by acknowledging how much courage this took and asking Tom to share what he learned rather than focusing on whether he enjoyed it or made friends immediately.

Sarah learned that celebrating these victories required being specific about what she was acknowledging. Instead of general praise like "I'm proud of you," she would say "I noticed you stayed and talked with that new person at the photography meeting even though I could see you were nervous. That took real courage."

This specific acknowledgment helped Tom recognize his own progress and build confidence in his ability to handle social challenges. Over time, Tom began celebrating his own small victories rather than only focusing on his social failures and anxieties.

The Quiet Strength of Gradual Growth

Avoidant personality disorder requires a fundamentally different approach to relationship building than other personality disorders. Success isn't measured in dramatic breakthroughs but in quiet moments of courage—a hand extended in greeting, an opinion shared despite fear of judgment, a social invitation accepted despite overwhelming anxiety.

Your role as a partner involves becoming a safe harbor from which your loved one can venture into the social world they both fear and crave. This means providing consistent reassurance without enabling complete withdrawal, encouraging growth without demanding performance, and celebrating progress that others might not even notice.

The journey with avoidant personality disorder is slow and requires enormous patience from both partners. But the rewards—watching someone who has lived in fear gradually develop confidence, seeing them discover that they are worthy of love and friendship, witnessing their world expand from isolation to connection—make the careful, gradual process worthwhile.

Progress happens not through dramatic confrontations with fear but through accumulating positive experiences that slowly rewire a brain convinced that social connection leads inevitably to pain. Your steady presence and gentle encouragement provide the foundation for this rewiring to occur.

Key Insights for Partners

- Fear of rejection in avoidant personality disorder is physically and emotionally overwhelming, not just ordinary social anxiety

- Building safety requires predictable, non-threatening interactions and explicit reassurance about your continued love and acceptance

- Supporting growth means encouraging small social risks rather than protecting your partner from all challenging situations

- Social events require preparation, escape planning, and recognition that your presence provides crucial security

- Progress happens in tiny increments that represent enormous courage and deserve specific, thoughtful acknowledgment

- Success is measured not in social performance but in gradual expansion of your partner's willingness to risk connection with others

Chapter 12: Dependent Personality Disorder

The Clinging Vine

Your phone buzzes for the fifteenth time this morning. Each text from your partner contains another question that most adults handle independently—what to wear to work, which route to take to avoid traffic, what to order for lunch. By afternoon, they're calling to ask if they should stay late to finish a project or leave on time, then calling again to confirm that you really meant what you said the first time. You love their trust in your judgment, but somewhere along the way, you became responsible for living two lives—yours and theirs.

When "I Need You" Becomes Suffocating

According to Bridges to Recovery research, dependent personality disorder creates one of the most emotionally challenging dynamics for partners because it transforms natural caregiving instincts into overwhelming responsibility for another adult's daily functioning. Your partner genuinely cannot make decisions independently—not because they lack intelligence or capability, but because their sense of self-worth and security depends entirely on having someone else take responsibility for their choices.

The research shows that people with dependent personality disorder experience genuine panic when faced with decisions, even minor ones. Their brain interprets independent choice-making as dangerous territory that could lead to mistakes, criticism, and ultimately abandonment by the people they depend on for emotional survival. This isn't manipulation or laziness—it's a learned survival mechanism that developed in response to early experiences where independence was punished or where caregivers provided inconsistent or conditional love.

How Dependency Manifests in Relationships:

Decision Paralysis: Your partner cannot choose what to wear, what to eat, which route to take, or what to watch on television without your input and approval. Even decisions they make independently require your validation afterward.

Constant Communication: They need to check in with you throughout the day, not just to share experiences but to get permission and approval for their actions and thoughts.

Emotional Regulation Through Others: Your partner's mood depends entirely on your mood and your availability. When you're happy and attentive, they feel secure. When you're busy, stressed, or need space, they become anxious and dysregulated.

Inability to Be Alone: They may call in sick to work when you travel, become physically ill when separated from you, or make elaborate arrangements to avoid being alone for extended periods.

Sacrifice of Personal Preferences: They consistently defer to your choices, often to the point where you don't know what they actually like or want because they've never developed independent preferences.

Crisis During Separations: Business trips, family obligations, or any situation that requires them to function independently creates genuine crisis and panic rather than normal missing-you feelings.

Case Example 1: Michael's Transformation from Caregiver to Partner Michael met Janet when they both worked at the same company. Janet seemed sweet and considerate, always asking for his advice about work projects and seeming to value his opinions highly. Michael felt flattered that someone would seek his guidance so consistently and interpreted Janet's dependence as respect for his intelligence and experience.

After they moved in together, Michael realized that Janet's advice-seeking extended to every aspect of daily life. She would ask Michael what to make for breakfast, what clothes to wear for different weather conditions, and even what television shows she should watch while he was at work. Janet couldn't make these decisions independently and would become anxious and indecisive when Michael suggested she choose for herself.

Michael initially found Janet's dependence endearing and felt needed and appreciated. But gradually, the constant responsibility for two people's lives became exhausting. Michael couldn't have a sick day without fielding calls from Janet about whether she should eat the leftovers in the refrigerator or order takeout. He couldn't work late without detailed instructions about what Janet should do with her evening.

The breaking point came when Michael had to attend his father's funeral in another state. Janet couldn't handle Michael being away during a crisis and made the trip about her needs rather than Michael's grief. Janet called Michael every few hours, crying about how scared she was alone and begging him to come home early. Michael realized he was spending his father's funeral managing Janet's anxiety instead of processing his own loss.

Michael recognized that his caretaking, while well-intentioned, had prevented Janet from developing her own coping skills and decision-making abilities. With professional help, Michael learned to support Janet's growth toward independence rather than enabling her dependency.

Breaking the Rescuer-Victim Cycle

According to research from Asteroidhealth, dependent personality disorder relationships often fall into a rescuer-victim cycle where one partner consistently saves the other from the consequences of their inability to function independently. This cycle feels like love and support but actually prevents the dependent partner from developing necessary life skills while exhausting the caregiving partner.

The Rescuer-Victim Cycle Looks Like:

Crisis Creation: The dependent partner faces situations that require independent decision-making or problem-solving and becomes overwhelmed, creating crisis situations that demand immediate rescue.

Rescue Response: The caregiving partner steps in to solve the problem, make the decision, or provide the emotional support needed to manage the crisis.

Temporary Relief: Both partners feel better temporarily—the dependent partner feels safe and cared for, while the rescuing partner feels needed and helpful.

Increased Dependency: The rescue reinforces the dependent partner's belief that they cannot handle challenges independently and increases their reliance on their partner for basic functioning.

Caregiver Exhaustion: The rescuing partner becomes increasingly overwhelmed by the responsibility of managing two lives but feels guilty about setting boundaries because their partner seems genuinely unable to cope.

Resentment and Guilt: The caregiving partner begins to feel resentful about the one-sided responsibility but feels guilty about these feelings because their partner's distress seems genuine and overwhelming.

Breaking this cycle requires the caregiving partner to stop rescuing while providing support for their partner's development of independent skills. This feels cruel initially because the dependent partner's distress is genuine, but rescue behaviors actually prevent the growth that would reduce their distress long-term.

Strategies for Breaking the Cycle:

Gradual Responsibility Transfer: Start with small decisions and gradually increase your partner's responsibility for their own choices rather than suddenly withdrawing all support.

Emotional Support Without Problem-Solving: Provide comfort and encouragement when your partner faces challenges but resist the urge to solve problems for them.

Consequence Tolerance: Allow your partner to experience the natural consequences of their decisions (both positive and negative) rather than protecting them from all discomfort.

Skill Teaching Rather Than Doing: Show your partner how to research decisions, weigh options, and problem-solve rather than providing ready-made solutions.

Boundary Setting with Compassion: Establish limits on your availability for decision-making and crisis management while reassuring your partner that boundaries don't mean abandonment.

Teaching Independence Without Abandonment

The most delicate aspect of dependent personality disorder relationships involves encouraging independence while maintaining the emotional security your partner needs to feel safe enough to try functioning on their own. According to Avalon Malibu research, this process requires careful balance between pushing for growth and providing enough support to prevent overwhelming anxiety that could trigger even more dependent behaviors.

Building Independence Gradually:

Start with Low-Stakes Decisions: Begin with choices that don't have serious consequences—what to have for lunch, which movie to watch, what to wear on casual days. Success with small decisions builds confidence for larger ones.

Create Decision-Making Frameworks: Teach your partner structured ways to approach choices: identify options, consider pros and cons, make a decision, and evaluate the outcome. This reduces the overwhelming feeling of not knowing how to choose.

Practice Tolerating Uncertainty: Help your partner learn that most decisions don't have perfect answers and that making adequate choices is sufficient. Perfectionism often paralyzes dependent personalities.

Celebrate Independent Choices: Acknowledge when your partner makes decisions on their own, regardless of the outcome. "I noticed you chose the restaurant for tonight—how did that feel?" reinforces their growing independence.

Provide Emotional Support During Growth: Recognize that learning independence feels scary and lonely for someone with dependent personality disorder. Offer comfort and encouragement while maintaining boundaries about decision-making responsibility.

Case Example 2: Sarah's Journey Toward Self-Reliance David watched his girlfriend Sarah struggle with simple daily decisions for the first year of their relationship. Sarah would call David multiple times during his workday to ask about everything from whether she should take an umbrella to what she should say in response to work emails. David initially provided detailed guidance for each question, thinking he was being supportive.

David realized that his constant advice-giving was preventing Sarah from developing her own judgment and decision-making skills. With guidance from a therapist, David began changing his approach to Sarah's requests for help.

Instead of telling Sarah what to do, David started asking questions that helped her think through decisions: "What do you think would happen if you chose option A versus option B?" or "What feels right to you when you think about it?" Initially, Sarah found these questions frustrating because she wanted definitive answers, but gradually she began developing her own decision-making process.

David also started setting boundaries around his availability for consultation. He let Sarah know that he wouldn't be available for decision-making calls during work hours but would discuss any important decisions when he got home. This forced Sarah to make some choices independently and to wait for discussion about others rather than getting immediate rescue.

Most importantly, David learned to celebrate Sarah's independent choices even when they weren't the decisions he would have made. When Sarah chose a restaurant he didn't particularly like, David focused on praising her decision-making process rather than critiquing her choice. This helped Sarah build confidence in her ability to make adequate decisions even if they weren't perfect.

Managing Decision Fatigue

Living with someone who has dependent personality disorder creates decision fatigue for the caregiving partner—the mental exhaustion that comes from being responsible for countless daily choices for two people. This fatigue affects your ability to make good decisions for yourself and can lead to resentment about the relationship dynamic.

Signs of Decision Fatigue:

Irritability About Small Requests: Finding yourself snapping at your partner for asking seemingly simple questions that you used to answer patiently.

Avoidance of Your Own Decisions: Putting off personal choices or decisions because your mental energy is depleted from managing your partner's choices.

Simplified Thinking: Making increasingly quick, black-and-white decisions rather than considering options carefully because you're too tired for complex analysis.

Physical Exhaustion: Feeling drained by conversations that involve multiple questions and requests for guidance, even about minor matters.

Resentment: Feeling angry that you can't have a conversation or activity without fielding questions about unrelated decisions your partner needs to make.

Strategies for Managing Decision Fatigue:

Batch Decision-Making Time: Set aside specific times when you're available to help with decisions rather than responding to requests throughout the day.

Limit Daily Decision Requests: Establish a reasonable number of decisions you'll help with each day and encourage your partner to prioritize their most important questions.

Encourage Independent Research: Ask your partner to gather information and present options before asking for your input rather than expecting you to do all the research.

Use Decision-Making Tools: Teach your partner to use pros-and-cons lists, decision matrices, or other structured approaches that reduce the emotional overwhelm of choice-making.

Protect Your Own Decision Energy: Make sure you're not depleting all your mental energy on your partner's choices while neglecting your own important decisions.

Creating Healthy Interdependence

The goal in dependent personality disorder relationships isn't complete independence—healthy relationships involve mutual dependence where both partners rely on each other for different types of support. According to Marriage.com research, the key is creating interdependence where dependency flows in both directions and both partners maintain their individual identities and capabilities.

Healthy Interdependence Characteristics:

Mutual Support: Both partners provide support for different challenges and decisions rather than all support flowing in one direction.

Maintained Individual Skills: Each partner retains the ability to function independently when necessary, even if they prefer to consult with each other.

Emotional Reciprocity: Both partners provide comfort, encouragement, and emotional support during difficult times rather than one person always being the giver.

Shared Decision-Making: Major decisions affecting both partners are made together, while personal decisions remain individual responsibilities.

Complementary Strengths: Partners rely on each other's different strengths and expertise rather than one partner being responsible for all types of decisions.

Building Toward Interdependence:

Identify Your Partner's Strengths: Help your partner recognize areas where they have good judgment or skills, and begin relying on their expertise in those areas.

Share Your Own Vulnerabilities: Let your partner see areas where you need support or guidance, creating opportunities for them to provide care and advice.

Create Reciprocal Consulting: Establish patterns where you ask your partner for input on decisions in their areas of strength or interest.

Maintain Individual Responsibilities: Ensure that each partner has some decisions and responsibilities that belong entirely to them.

Practice Temporary Separations: Build confidence through brief periods apart where each partner manages their own decisions and daily functioning.

Case Example 3: Building Balance in Daily Life Jennifer and Mark worked together to create healthier interdependence after recognizing that their relationship had become a one-way caretaking arrangement. Mark had dependent personality disorder and had become reliant on Jennifer for virtually all decisions, while Jennifer felt overwhelmed by the constant responsibility.

Jennifer started by identifying areas where Mark actually had good judgment and expertise. Mark was knowledgeable about technology and had excellent research skills, so Jennifer began asking for his advice about electronics purchases and online services. This gave Mark opportunities to be helpful rather than always being the one needing help.

Jennifer also began sharing some of her own decision-making challenges with Mark. Instead of handling all household management independently, Jennifer asked Mark to research options for home repairs, insurance changes, or major purchases. This created opportunities for Mark to contribute to their shared life rather than just receiving Jennifer's care.

Most importantly, Jennifer established areas of individual responsibility for both partners. Mark became responsible for his own schedule management, personal health appointments, and social plans with his own friends. Jennifer stopped monitoring these areas and allowed Mark to succeed or struggle with the consequences of his own choices.

Over time, this approach helped Mark develop confidence in his decision-making abilities while reducing Jennifer's sense of overwhelming responsibility. Their relationship became more balanced, with both partners contributing different types of support and expertise rather than Jennifer being the sole decision-maker and caregiver.

The Delicate Balance of Growing Together

Dependent personality disorder relationships require extraordinary patience and careful attention to the balance between support and enablement. Your partner's need for guidance and reassurance is genuine, but meeting every need prevents the growth that would ultimately reduce their anxiety and increase their confidence.

Success in these relationships means learning to love someone enough to let them struggle sometimes, to provide emotional support while maintaining boundaries about decision-making responsibility, and to celebrate small steps toward independence even when progress feels painfully slow.

The reward for this careful balance is watching someone who has lived in fear of their own choices gradually discover their capacity for good judgment and independent functioning. The process requires enormous patience from both partners but ultimately creates a stronger, more balanced relationship where both people contribute to their shared life.

Your role is not to be your partner's decision-maker for life but to provide the security and support they need while they develop the skills and confidence to manage their own choices. This delicate process transforms relationships from caregiver-patient dynamics into genuine partnerships between capable adults.

Key Insights for Partners

- Dependency in personality disorder stems from genuine panic about decision-making rather than laziness or manipulation

- The rescuer-victim cycle prevents growth by reinforcing the dependent partner's belief that they cannot function independently

- Teaching independence requires gradual responsibility transfer with emotional support but without problem-solving rescue

- Decision fatigue affects caregiving partners and requires boundaries around availability and energy allocation

- Healthy interdependence involves mutual support and shared strengths rather than one-way caretaking arrangements

- Progress toward independence is slow and requires celebrating small victories while maintaining supportive boundaries

Chapter 13: Obsessive-Compulsive Personality Disorder

Living by the Rules

Your partner spends three hours organizing the closet by color, season, and frequency of wear, then becomes genuinely distressed when you hang a shirt in the wrong section. They work until midnight perfecting a presentation that was already excellent at 6 PM, missing dinner and your attempt at conversation because "it's not quite right yet." You've learned to check your own standards at the door—nothing you do will meet their exacting requirements, and their need for perfection has somehow become a judgment on your more relaxed approach to life.

Perfectionism vs Love: When Nothing is Ever Good Enough

Obsessive-compulsive personality disorder transforms relationships into constant performance evaluations where love gets measured by adherence to impossibly high standards. Your partner doesn't just prefer things done well—they need things done perfectly, and their definition of perfect often changes based on circumstances, mood, or new information they've discovered about the "right" way to handle various situations.

This isn't the same as being detail-oriented or having high standards. People with OCPD experience genuine distress when things don't meet their internal criteria for correctness. Their brain interprets imperfection as moral failure, and they extend this same standard to everyone around them. Your casual approach to household organization isn't just different from theirs—in their mind, it's wrong, and your willingness to accept "good enough" reflects poorly on your character and commitment.

How Perfectionism Affects Relationships:

Criticism Disguised as Help: Your partner points out flaws in your work, appearance, or methods under the guise of helping you improve, but the constant corrections feel more like judgment than support.

Rigid Standards for Affection: Love gets demonstrated through meeting their standards rather than through emotional connection. If you don't load the dishwasher correctly, it means you don't care about their needs.

Process Over Outcome: Your partner becomes so focused on doing things the "right way" that they lose sight of the purpose of activities. A romantic dinner gets ruined because the table settings aren't perfect.

Emotional Distance Through Tasks: Instead of connecting through conversation or physical affection, your partner shows love through organizing, fixing, or improving things around you.

Resentment About Standards: You begin to feel like you can never do anything well enough, while your partner feels frustrated that you don't appreciate their efforts to maintain quality and order.

The Workaholic Partner: Competing with Achievement

According to research from Asteroidhealth and MedCircle, people with OCPD often become so absorbed in work and achievement that their relationships suffer from neglect. This isn't ordinary career ambition—it's a compulsive need to demonstrate worth through productivity and perfection that makes it nearly impossible for them to relax, enjoy leisure time, or be emotionally present with loved ones.

Your partner might work late every night not because their job requires it, but because they can't stop refining and perfecting their work until it meets their internal standards. They might spend weekends organizing files, updating systems, or researching better ways to handle professional tasks rather than spending time with you or pursuing enjoyable activities together.

Work Addiction vs Career Success:

Inability to Delegate: Your partner must personally handle tasks that others could manage because they don't trust anyone else to meet their standards.

Endless Revision: Projects that could be completed adequately in reasonable time become ongoing perfectionist pursuits that consume evenings and weekends.

Guilt About Leisure: Your partner feels uncomfortable with relaxation or entertainment, viewing these activities as lazy or unproductive rather than necessary for mental health.

Identity Through Productivity: Your partner's self-worth depends entirely on their work output and achievement rather than their relationships or personal qualities.

Anxiety About Standards: They worry constantly about whether their work is good enough, often seeking excessive feedback and validation from supervisors or colleagues.

Case Example 1: Susan's Journey from Rigidity to Flexibility David married Susan partly because he admired her attention to detail and high standards. Susan was successful at work, maintained a beautifully organized home, and seemed to approach everything with thoughtfulness and care. David initially appreciated living in a well-organized environment and felt proud of Susan's professional accomplishments.

Over time, David realized that Susan's standards weren't just high— they were inflexible and all-consuming. Susan would spend hours perfecting work presentations that were already excellent, missing social events and family gatherings because the work "wasn't ready yet." Susan couldn't enjoy vacations because she worried about work piling up and couldn't relax without feeling guilty about being unproductive.

At home, Susan's need for perfection extended to every aspect of their shared life. David couldn't load the dishwasher without Susan rearranging it to meet her standards. Their social calendar became Susan's responsibility because she couldn't trust David to plan events that would meet her criteria for success. Even David's attempts to help with household tasks would be redone by Susan because they weren't completed to her specifications.

The breaking point came when Susan spent their anniversary evening organizing their financial files instead of celebrating their relationship. When David expressed hurt about this choice, Susan became defensive, explaining that their financial organization was more important than "wasting time" on romantic gestures they couldn't afford if their finances weren't properly managed.

With professional help, Susan learned to recognize how her perfectionism was affecting her relationships and her own well-being. Susan worked on accepting "good enough" in non-critical areas and scheduling specific times for organizing and perfecting tasks rather than allowing these needs to consume all her free time.

Practical Negotiations for Daily Life

Living successfully with someone who has OCPD requires ongoing negotiation about standards, processes, and priorities. You can't simply ignore their need for order and perfection, but you also can't allow their standards to completely dictate your shared life. The key lies in finding compromises that respect both your need for flexibility and their need for structure.

Areas Requiring Negotiation:

Household Organization: Agree on which areas need to meet their high standards and which areas can be managed more casually. Perhaps the kitchen must be perfectly organized, but the garage can be functional without being pristine.

Social Commitments: Establish limits on how much preparation and perfection are required for social events. Your partner might need detailed planning, but you need reasonable limits on preparation time.

Work-Life Balance: Set boundaries about work time that protect time for your relationship and shared activities. Your partner needs structure, but your relationship needs attention too.

Decision-Making Processes: Agree on how much research and analysis are appropriate for different types of decisions. Major purchases might warrant extensive research, but dinner choices don't need comparison shopping.

Quality Standards: Identify which tasks truly benefit from perfectionist attention and which can be handled adequately with less intensive effort.

Compromise Strategies:

The 80% Rule: Agree that most tasks only need to be 80% perfect unless there are specific reasons why higher standards are necessary.

Time Limits: Set maximum time limits for perfectionist activities. Your partner can organize or refine tasks within agreed timeframes, but must stop when time expires.

Division of Responsibilities: Let your partner maintain perfectionist control over areas that matter most to them while you handle other areas according to your own standards.

Scheduled Perfection Time: Designate specific times for organizing, refining, and perfecting tasks rather than allowing these activities to interrupt all other plans.

Priority Systems: Help your partner identify which perfectionist activities are most important and focus their energy on those rather than applying the same standards to everything.

OCPD vs OCD: Critical Differences That Matter

According to WebMD and other medical sources, obsessive-compulsive personality disorder (OCPD) is frequently confused with obsessive-compulsive disorder (OCD), but these are distinct conditions that require different approaches in relationships. Understanding the difference affects how you respond to your partner's behaviors and what kind of professional help might be most beneficial.

Key Differences Between OCPD and OCD:

Ego-Syntonic vs Ego-Dystonic: People with OCPD believe their perfectionist behaviors and rigid standards are correct and necessary. People with OCD recognize that their compulsions are excessive and unwanted but feel unable to control them.

Flexibility vs Compulsion: OCPD involves rigid adherence to personal standards and ways of doing things. OCD involves specific compulsions that must be performed to reduce anxiety, often involving repetitive behaviors or mental rituals.

Pride vs Distress: People with OCPD often take pride in their high standards and organizational skills. People with OCD typically feel distressed and embarrassed about their compulsive behaviors.

Broad vs Specific: OCPD affects general life patterns around perfectionism, control, and order. OCD typically involves specific obsessions and compulsions that may not affect other areas of life.

Treatment Approaches: OCPD often benefits from therapy focused on flexibility and relationship skills. OCD typically requires specialized treatment for anxiety and compulsive behaviors.

Why the Distinction Matters for Partners:

Different Validation Needs: OCPD partners may need acknowledgment of their positive qualities (organization, thoroughness, reliability) while working on flexibility. OCD partners need support in recognizing that their compulsions are symptoms rather than personality traits.

Different Boundary Strategies: With OCPD, you might negotiate about standards and processes. With OCD, you might need to avoid enabling compulsions while providing emotional support for anxiety.

Different Professional Help: OCPD benefits from therapy that addresses personality patterns and relationship dynamics. OCD often requires specialized anxiety treatment and possibly medication.

Case Example 2: Recognizing the Difference in Treatment Maria initially thought her husband Carlos had OCD because of his rigid routines and need for things to be done in specific ways. Carlos would become very upset if their morning routine varied or if Maria changed the organization system he had established for their home. Maria tried to accommodate Carlos by following his routines exactly and avoiding any changes that might trigger his anxiety.

But Carlos wasn't experiencing the distress and recognition of irrationality that characterizes OCD. Instead, Carlos believed his systems were superior and became frustrated when Maria didn't appreciate the efficiency and logic of his approaches. Carlos took pride in his organizational skills and saw Maria's more flexible approach as careless rather than simply different.

When Carlos finally agreed to therapy, the therapist helped Maria understand that Carlos had OCPD rather than OCD. This distinction changed Maria's approach significantly. Instead of trying to prevent Carlos's anxiety by accommodating all his systems, Maria learned to negotiate about which systems were truly necessary and which represented Carlos's preferences rather than needs.

Maria also learned to appreciate Carlos's genuine strengths—his reliability, attention to detail, and ability to manage complex organizational tasks—while maintaining boundaries about areas where his perfectionism interfered with their relationship or her own well-being.

Making Space for Spontaneity and Joy

One of the greatest challenges in OCPD relationships is maintaining space for spontaneity, fun, and emotional connection when your partner's need for control and perfection tends to dominate daily life. People with OCPD often struggle to enjoy activities that don't have productive outcomes, making it difficult to maintain the playful, relaxed interactions that keep relationships emotionally connected.

Strategies for Creating Balance:

Schedule Spontaneity: This sounds contradictory, but people with OCPD often need structure even around relaxation. Set aside time for unstructured activities rather than expecting spontaneous fun to happen naturally.

Lower-Stakes Fun: Choose activities that don't trigger your partner's perfectionist tendencies. A casual walk might work better than a elaborate dinner party that requires extensive planning and preparation.

Appreciate Their Version of Fun: Your OCPD partner might genuinely enjoy organizing activities or researching topics of interest. Find ways to connect around their interests rather than expecting them to adopt your more spontaneous approach to entertainment.

Protect Emotional Connection Time: Establish periods when work, organizing, and perfectionist activities are off-limits so you can focus on your relationship and emotional intimacy.

Model Flexible Thinking: Demonstrate through your own behavior that things can be enjoyable and successful even when they're not perfect, without directly criticizing your partner's standards.

Case Example 3: Finding Joy in Structure Jennifer learned to work with rather than against her boyfriend Mark's OCPD tendencies when planning enjoyable activities together. Initially, Jennifer would try to surprise Mark with spontaneous outings or unplanned adventures, which invariably created anxiety and conflict because Mark couldn't enjoy activities that weren't properly planned and organized.

Jennifer discovered that Mark could enjoy spontaneous activities if she provided enough structure around the spontaneity. Instead of suggesting "Let's just drive somewhere and see what we find," Jennifer learned to say "Let's plan a Saturday afternoon for exploring—we can research three possible destinations and choose one when we get in the car."

Jennifer also learned to appreciate Mark's version of enjoyable activities. Mark genuinely found pleasure in organizing their photo albums, researching vacation destinations, and creating efficient systems for household management. Instead of viewing these activities as work that prevented fun, Jennifer learned to participate in ways that felt connecting rather than burdensome.

Most importantly, Jennifer established boundaries around when perfectionist activities could occur. Mark could spend Sunday mornings organizing and planning, but Saturday evenings were reserved for relaxation and connection without any productivity requirements. This structure gave Mark the control and organization time he needed while protecting space for their relationship to flourish.

The Art of Loving Someone Who Lives by Rules

OCPD relationships can be deeply rewarding when both partners learn to appreciate the benefits of structure and high standards while maintaining space for flexibility and emotional connection. Your partner's attention to detail, reliability, and commitment to excellence can provide security and stability that many relationships lack.

The challenge lies in helping your partner understand that relationships thrive on emotional connection rather than perfect performance, and that love isn't demonstrated through meeting impossible standards but through mutual care, respect, and acceptance of each other's different approaches to life.

Success requires patience with your partner's need for control and perfection while maintaining boundaries that protect your own well-being and the spontaneous, imperfect moments that make relationships joyful. This means learning to negotiate rather than accommodate completely, and to appreciate your partner's strengths while addressing the ways their rigidity interferes with intimacy.

The goal isn't to eliminate your partner's high standards but to create space for both excellence and imperfection, both structure and spontaneity, both productivity and play within your shared life together.

Key Insights for Partners

- OCPD perfectionism stems from genuine distress about imperfection rather than simple preference for high standards

- Work addiction in OCPD reflects compulsive productivity needs that compete with relationship time and emotional availability

- Daily life requires ongoing negotiation about standards, processes, and priorities that respect both partners' needs

- OCPD differs from OCD in that people take pride in their rigid standards rather than experiencing distress about compulsive behaviors

- Creating space for spontaneity and joy requires structure and planning that accommodate rather than eliminate perfectionist tendencies

- Success involves appreciating your partner's genuine strengths while maintaining boundaries that protect emotional connection and flexibility

Chapter 14: Therapeutic Interventions That Actually Work

The therapy landscape for personality disorder relationships resembles a confusing maze of acronyms, theoretical approaches, and conflicting advice. You've probably heard recommendations for everything from individual therapy to couples counseling, from meditation apps to intensive retreats. The challenge isn't finding therapy—it's finding therapy that actually works for the specific dynamics created by personality disorders. Not all therapeutic approaches are created equal, and some can actually make personality disorder relationships worse rather than better.

DBT for Partners

Skills That Save Relationships

Dialectical Behavior Therapy (DBT) wasn't designed specifically for partners of people with personality disorders, but according to Psychology Today research, it provides some of the most practical and effective tools for surviving and thriving in these challenging relationships. DBT teaches concrete skills that help you manage emotional reactivity, communicate effectively during crises, and maintain your own mental health while supporting someone with a personality disorder.

The beauty of DBT lies in its practical, skill-based approach. Instead of spending years analyzing why you feel overwhelmed by your partner's behaviors, DBT teaches you what to do when you feel overwhelmed. Instead of exploring childhood roots of codependency, DBT gives you specific techniques for maintaining boundaries while still being supportive.

The Four Core DBT Modules for Partners:

Distress Tolerance Skills: These help you survive crisis situations without making them worse through your own emotional reactions. Your partner's personality disorder will create periodic crises—emotional meltdowns, threats, accusations, or other intense situations. Your ability to stay grounded during these crises often determines the outcome.

The STOP skill becomes essential during personality disorder crises. Stop what you're doing, take a breath, observe what's actually happening versus what emotions are making it feel like, and proceed with intention rather than reaction. This simple framework prevents you from getting swept into your partner's emotional storm and making impulsive decisions you'll regret later.

Distraction techniques help you manage your own emotional overload when your partner's behaviors trigger intense reactions in you. Instead of ruminating about their accusations or trying to fix their emotional state, you redirect your attention to activities that restore your emotional balance.

Emotion Regulation Skills: Living with personality disorder dynamics often creates secondary trauma in partners. You might develop hypervigilance, anxiety, depression, or other emotional responses that interfere with your ability to think clearly and make good decisions about your relationship.

The PLEASE skill addresses the foundation of emotional regulation—treating physical illness, balancing eating, avoiding mood-altering substances, balancing sleep, and getting exercise. Personality disorder relationships are stressful, and stress affects your physical health, which affects your emotional stability.

Opposite action helps when your emotions don't fit the facts of situations. If your partner with avoidant personality disorder withdraws after an argument, your emotional impulse might be to pursue and reassure them. But if pursuing typically makes their withdrawal worse, opposite action would be giving them space while remaining emotionally available.

Interpersonal Effectiveness Skills: These skills help you get your needs met and maintain your boundaries while staying connected to your partner. Personality disorders often involve communication patterns that make normal relationship skills ineffective.

The DEAR MAN skill provides a framework for making requests or setting boundaries clearly. Describe the situation, express your feelings, assert your needs, reinforce positive outcomes, stay mindful of your goal, appear confident, and negotiate when possible. This structure helps you communicate effectively even when your partner's responses are intense or unreasonable.

Mindfulness Skills: These help you stay present and maintain perspective during the emotional intensity of personality disorder relationships. Mindfulness isn't about becoming zen or detached — it's about staying aware of your own experience and choices rather than getting lost in your partner's emotional chaos.

Case Example 1: Sarah's DBT Transformation Sarah's relationship with Mark, who had borderline personality disorder, was consuming her life. She would spend hours every day managing Mark's emotional crises, trying to reassure him about imagined threats to their relationship, and walking on eggshells to avoid triggering his abandonment fears. Sarah developed anxiety and depression from the constant stress and began to lose her sense of identity outside of Mark's needs.

Sarah learned DBT skills in individual therapy and immediately began applying them to her relationship challenges. When Mark accused

Sarah of planning to leave him (triggered by her working late one evening), Sarah used the STOP skill instead of her usual pattern of providing detailed explanations and reassurances.

Sarah stopped defending herself against the accusation, took a breath to notice her own emotional state, observed that Mark was in an emotional crisis that wasn't based on actual evidence, and proceeded by acknowledging Mark's fear without accepting responsibility for managing it. "I can see you're scared I might leave. That must feel awful. I'm not planning to leave, and I'm going to give you some space to calm down."

This approach helped de-escalate the situation more quickly than Sarah's previous attempts to reason with Mark during his emotional storms. More importantly, it helped Sarah maintain her own emotional balance instead of getting swept into Mark's crisis.

Sarah also used interpersonal effectiveness skills to set boundaries about her availability for crisis management. Using DEAR MAN, Sarah explained that she could provide emotional support for one major crisis conversation per day, but wouldn't engage in multiple crisis discussions about the same issue. This boundary helped Mark learn to manage his emotions between their conversations instead of relying on constant reassurance.

Schema Therapy: Rewiring Destructive Patterns

According to Psychology Today research, Schema Therapy addresses the deep-rooted patterns that drive personality disorder behaviors by focusing on "schemas"—core beliefs about yourself, others, and relationships that develop early in life and influence all future relationships. For partners, understanding schema therapy concepts helps explain why logical arguments and surface-level changes don't resolve personality disorder patterns.

Schemas are like mental templates that filter how we interpret experiences. Someone who developed an "abandonment schema" will interpret neutral relationship events as signs of impending abandonment. Someone with a "defectiveness schema" will assume that if you really knew them, you would reject them. These schemas operate automatically and influence behavior even when the person recognizes that their fears aren't logical.

Common Schemas in Personality Disorders:

Abandonment Schema: The belief that important people will inevitably leave or become unavailable. This drives clingy, possessive, or testing behaviors designed to prevent abandonment.

Mistrust/Abuse Schema: The expectation that others will hurt, manipulate, or take advantage of you. This creates hypervigilance and defensive behaviors that push people away.

Defectiveness Schema: The belief that you are fundamentally flawed and unworthy of love. This drives perfectionism, people-pleasing, or defensive superiority as attempts to hide perceived inadequacies.

Dependence Schema: The belief that you cannot handle life's challenges independently. This creates excessive reliance on others for decision-making and emotional regulation.

Entitlement Schema: The belief that you are special and deserve special treatment. This drives demanding, controlling, or exploitative behaviors.

Understanding these schemas helps partners recognize that personality disorder behaviors aren't really about you or your relationship—they're about deeply held beliefs that your partner developed long before they met you.

Case Example 2: Understanding Tom's Schema Patterns Lisa's husband Tom had narcissistic personality disorder, and Lisa struggled to understand why Tom would become enraged by seemingly minor events—like Lisa receiving a compliment at a party or Lisa's friend getting a promotion at work. Tom would interpret these neutral events as threats to his status and would spend days criticizing Lisa or her friends to restore his sense of superiority.

Learning about schema therapy helped Lisa understand that Tom operated from a "grandiosity schema" that required him to see himself as special and superior to others. This wasn't conscious arrogance—it was a defensive strategy Tom's mind used to protect him from feeling inadequate and worthless, which were the feelings underneath his grandiose presentation.

Lisa realized that Tom's criticism of her achievements wasn't really about her—it was about his need to maintain his schema that he was the most successful and important person in their relationship. This understanding didn't excuse Tom's behavior, but it helped Lisa stop taking his reactions personally and recognize that his responses came from his internal struggles rather than actual problems with her choices or achievements.

Lisa learned to respond to Tom's schema-driven behaviors differently. Instead of defending her accomplishments or trying to reassure Tom about his own worth, Lisa would acknowledge Tom's feelings without engaging with the content of his criticisms. "I can see you're feeling uncomfortable about something. That sounds difficult for you." This approach avoided triggering Tom's defensive responses while not enabling his critical behaviors.

Mentalization

The Magic of Understanding Minds

According to Cleveland Clinic research, mentalization-based therapy focuses on the ability to understand mental states—both your own and others'—that underlie behavior. Many personality disorders involve difficulties with mentalization, meaning your partner might struggle to understand their own emotions or to accurately read your intentions and mental states.

Mentalization is the skill of recognizing that behavior is driven by thoughts, feelings, beliefs, and intentions rather than being random or deliberately hurtful. When someone has good mentalization skills, they can think things like "She seems upset—maybe she's stressed about work" rather than "She's upset—she must be angry at me."

Poor mentalization leads to misinterpretations of others' behavior and inability to understand your own emotional reactions. Your partner might interpret your tiredness as rejection, your need for space as abandonment, or your different opinion as attack. They also might not understand their own emotional reactions, leading to confusion about why they feel overwhelmed or angry in certain situations.

How Mentalization Helps Relationships:

Reduces Emotional Reactivity: When you understand that behavior comes from mental states rather than being personal attacks, you react less defensively to your partner's personality disorder symptoms.

Improves Communication: You learn to share your mental states explicitly rather than expecting your partner to read your mind accurately, and you learn to ask about their mental states rather than assuming you know what they're thinking.

Increases Empathy: Understanding the mental states driving your partner's behavior helps you respond with compassion rather than anger, even when their behavior is problematic.

Builds Self-Awareness: You become better at recognizing your own mental states and how they influence your reactions to your partner's behaviors.

Case Example 3: Building Mentalization Skills Together David and Amanda both struggled with mentalization in their relationship. Amanda had borderline personality disorder and would frequently misinterpret David's mental states, assuming that his quiet moods meant he was angry with her or planning to leave. David would become frustrated with these misinterpretations and would withdraw further, confirming Amanda's fears.

David learned to make his mental states more explicit rather than expecting Amanda to read them accurately. Instead of being quietly tired after work, David would say, "I'm feeling drained from my day at work, but I'm happy to see you. I need about thirty minutes to decompress, and then I'd love to hear about your day."

Amanda learned to check her interpretations of David's behavior rather than assuming she knew what he was thinking. Instead of concluding that David's tiredness meant he was losing interest in their relationship, Amanda learned to ask, "I notice you seem quiet tonight. How are you feeling about us?" This gave David opportunities to clarify his mental state instead of having to defend against Amanda's misinterpretations.

Both partners learned to mentalize their own emotions during conflicts. Instead of Amanda saying, "You're making me feel abandoned," she learned to say, "When you withdraw, I start feeling scared that you don't want to be with me anymore." This helped David understand Amanda's mental state without feeling blamed for causing her emotions.

Finding the Right Therapist

(And Knowing When They're Wrong)

Not all therapists understand personality disorders, and some therapeutic approaches can actually make personality disorder relationships worse rather than better. Finding effective help requires knowing what to look for and being willing to change providers when therapy isn't helping.

Red Flags in Personality Disorder Therapy:

Therapist Takes Sides: Good therapy maintains neutrality and helps both partners understand their contributions to relationship problems rather than identifying one person as the victim and the other as the abuser.

Focus Only on Communication: While communication skills are helpful, personality disorders require more specialized approaches that address emotional regulation, trauma history, and ingrained patterns.

Pushing for Quick Reconciliation: Personality disorder relationships often need significant individual work before couples therapy can be effective. Therapists who rush into relationship repair without addressing underlying issues often make things worse.

Minimizing Safety Concerns: Any therapist who encourages you to stay in relationships where you feel unsafe or who minimizes abuse is not appropriate for personality disorder situations.

Lack of Personality Disorder Knowledge: If your therapist doesn't understand the specific challenges of personality disorders, they may provide generic relationship advice that doesn't apply to your situation.

What to Look for in Effective Therapy:

Specialized Training: Look for therapists trained in DBT, schema therapy, mentalization-based therapy, or other approaches specifically designed for personality disorders.

Individual Work First: Many effective approaches recommend individual therapy before or alongside couples therapy, allowing each partner to develop skills and stability.

Focus on Skills: Good personality disorder therapy teaches concrete skills for emotional regulation, communication, and boundary setting rather than just providing emotional support.

Realistic Expectations: Effective therapists help you understand that personality disorder changes happen slowly and require sustained effort from the person with the disorder.

Safety Assessment: Qualified therapists will assess for abuse, safety concerns, and whether the relationship is appropriate for therapeutic intervention.

Couples Therapy: When It Helps vs When It Harms

According to research from Talkspace and The Gottman Institute, couples therapy can be helpful for personality disorder relationships under specific circumstances, but it can also be harmful when applied incorrectly or at the wrong time. Understanding when couples therapy is appropriate and when it should be avoided can save you time, money, and potential additional relationship damage.

When Couples Therapy Can Help:

Both Partners Are Stable: When the person with the personality disorder is engaged in individual treatment and has developed basic emotional regulation skills, couples therapy can help address relationship patterns.

No Active Abuse: Couples therapy assumes both partners can safely express their needs and concerns. When abuse is present, couples therapy can actually make things worse by giving the abusive partner more tools for manipulation.

Motivation for Change: Both partners need to be willing to examine their own behaviors and make changes. If one partner attends therapy just to prove they're right, the process won't be successful.

Basic Safety Exists: Both partners need to feel emotionally and physically safe enough to be honest about their experiences and needs.

When Couples Therapy Can Harm:

Active Crisis or Instability: When the person with the personality disorder is in acute crisis, experiencing severe symptoms, or not engaged in individual treatment, couples therapy often escalates rather than resolves conflicts.

Presence of Abuse: Couples therapy with abusive partners often provides them with more sophisticated manipulation tools and can increase danger for the abused partner.

Severe Personality Disorders: Some personality disorders (particularly antisocial and severe narcissistic) may not be appropriate for couples therapy because the person lacks the empathy and motivation necessary for relationship change.

Therapist Incompetence: When therapists don't understand personality disorders, couples therapy can reinforce unhealthy dynamics rather than changing them.

Online Resources and Support Groups That Deliver

According to research from Emotions Matter and BPD Video communities, online resources can provide crucial support for partners dealing with personality disorder relationships, especially when local resources aren't available or when you need support outside of business hours.

Effective Online Resources:

Specialized Forums: Communities specifically for partners of people with specific personality disorders provide understanding and practical advice from people with similar experiences.

Educational Websites: Sites that provide accurate information about personality disorders, relationship dynamics, and coping strategies can help you understand what you're dealing with.

Virtual Support Groups: Online meetings allow you to connect with others without geographic limitations and often provide more scheduling flexibility than in-person groups.

Professional Online Therapy: Many qualified therapists now offer remote sessions, which can provide access to specialized care that might not be available in your area.

What to Avoid Online:

Generic Relationship Advice: Most relationship advice doesn't apply to personality disorder dynamics and can actually be harmful when applied to these situations.

Trauma Bonding Communities: Some online groups become focused on sharing war stories rather than developing healthy coping strategies or making positive changes.

Unmoderated Forums: Groups without professional oversight can sometimes provide dangerous advice or become dominated by people with their own untreated mental health issues.

Misinformation Sites: Be cautious of sites that demonize people with personality disorders or provide inaccurate information about these conditions.

The Foundation of Real Change

Effective therapy for personality disorder relationships requires specialized approaches that understand the unique challenges these conditions create. Generic relationship counseling or individual therapy that doesn't address personality disorder dynamics often fails to create meaningful change and can sometimes make situations worse.

The key to successful therapeutic intervention lies in finding providers who understand personality disorders, using evidence-based approaches that teach concrete skills, and maintaining realistic expectations about the pace and nature of change in these relationships.

Your therapeutic journey may involve multiple approaches—individual therapy to develop your own skills and heal from relationship trauma, specialized therapy for your partner if they're willing to engage, and possibly couples therapy once both partners have developed sufficient stability and skills to engage productively.

The investment in proper therapeutic support pays dividends not just in your current relationship, but in your ability to maintain healthy boundaries and relationships throughout your life. These skills become part of your toolkit for handling any future challenges with confidence and clarity.

Key Insights for Professional Support

- DBT provides practical skills for managing emotional reactivity, maintaining boundaries, and surviving crises common in personality disorder relationships

- Schema therapy helps partners understand the deep-rooted beliefs that drive personality disorder behaviors, reducing personal blame and increasing empathy

- Mentalization skills improve communication by helping partners understand the mental states behind behaviors rather than making assumptions

- Finding effective therapists requires seeking specialized training in personality disorders and avoiding providers who minimize safety concerns or rush relationship repair

- Couples therapy can help when both partners are stable and motivated, but can harm when abuse is present or during active crisis periods

- Online resources provide valuable support when chosen carefully, but generic relationship advice and unmoderated forums should be avoided

Chapter 15: The Art of Boundaries
- Your Survival Manual

You've tried being understanding, accommodating, and endlessly patient. You've adjusted your expectations, modified your behaviors, and bent over backward to avoid triggering your partner's personality disorder symptoms. But somewhere in all that accommodation, you lost yourself. Your needs became secondary, your feelings became inconvenient, and your own well-being became something you manage around the edges of someone else's mental health condition. This isn't love—it's self-erasure disguised as compassion.

Boundary Setting for Each Personality Disorder Type

Effective boundaries look different depending on which personality disorder you're dealing with because each condition creates unique challenges and manipulative patterns. Cookie-cutter boundary advice fails because it doesn't account for how different personality disorders will test, challenge, and attempt to circumvent your limits.

Paranoid Personality Disorder Boundaries:

With paranoid personalities, boundaries must be crystal clear and consistently maintained because any flexibility will be interpreted as evidence that your limits aren't genuine. Your partner's suspicious nature means they're constantly looking for proof that you're deceiving them, which makes boundary-setting feel like confirmation of their fears.

Set boundaries around surveillance behaviors explicitly. "I will share my location with you, but I won't provide detailed explanations for every interaction I have throughout the day." Then maintain this limit consistently, even when your partner becomes convinced that your boundary is proof of suspicious behavior.

Establish limits on accusation discussions. "I will listen to concerns you have about our relationship, but I won't participate in conversations that assume I'm lying or cheating." This prevents you from getting trapped in circular arguments designed to make you prove your innocence.

Schizoid Personality Disorder Boundaries:

With schizoid personalities, boundaries focus on preventing yourself from becoming their sole source of social connection while respecting their genuine need for emotional space. These boundaries protect you from isolation and relationship stagnation.

Set expectations about social participation. "I need us to maintain some shared social activities. You don't have to enjoy them, but I need you to participate occasionally rather than leaving me to handle all social obligations alone."

Create boundaries around emotional reciprocity. "I understand that emotional expression is difficult for you, but I need some acknowledgment of my feelings and experiences. You don't have to match my emotional intensity, but I need to know that you hear me."

Borderline Personality Disorder Boundaries:

With borderline personalities, boundaries must be maintained with exceptional consistency because any wavering will trigger testing behaviors designed to see if your limits are real. These boundaries often feel cruel because they involve not rescuing someone who appears to be genuinely suffering.

Establish crisis response limits. "I will help you during genuine emergencies, but I won't cancel my plans or responsibilities every time you feel overwhelmed. We need to develop a plan for managing your emotions that doesn't require my constant availability."

Set boundaries around relationship ultimatums. "I won't make permanent relationship decisions based on temporary emotional states. If you want to discuss our relationship, we can do that when you're calm, but threats and ultimatums won't influence my choices."

Narcissistic Personality Disorder Boundaries:

With narcissistic personalities, boundaries must be enforced without extensive explanation or justification because attempts to help them understand your limits will be used as opportunities for argument and manipulation.

Establish limits on criticism and devaluation. "I won't participate in conversations where you're insulting me or putting me down. If you want to discuss problems, we can do that respectfully, or we can take a break from talking."

Set boundaries around attention and admiration. "I care about your accomplishments and I want to celebrate your successes, but I won't provide constant validation or compete with others to make you feel special."

Case Example 1: Learning to Set Boundaries with Different Approaches Maria learned that the boundary-setting strategies she used with her previous partner (who had anxiety issues) were completely ineffective with her current partner Jake, who had narcissistic personality disorder. With her previous partner, gentle explanations and compromises had worked well. With Jake, these same approaches were interpreted as opportunities for negotiation and manipulation.

Maria's first attempt at boundary-setting involved explaining her needs in detail and asking Jake to understand her perspective. "I feel overwhelmed when you criticize my appearance and I need you to understand how that affects my self-esteem." Jake used this information to refine his criticism, making comments that were technically not about Maria's appearance but were equally damaging to her confidence.

Maria learned to set boundaries with Jake using minimal explanation and maximum consistency. Instead of explaining her emotional needs, Maria would simply state her limits and follow through. "I don't participate in conversations where you're putting me down," followed by leaving the room immediately when Jake began critical comments.

This approach was more effective because it didn't provide Jake with information he could use to circumvent the boundary, and it didn't require his understanding or agreement for Maria to protect herself.

Scripts That Work: What to Say and When

According to PeoplePsych research, specific language choices can make the difference between boundaries that hold and boundaries that crumble under pressure from personality disorder manipulation. The key lies in using language that's direct, non-negotiable, and doesn't invite argument or explanation.

Effective Boundary Scripts:

"I will..." vs "I need you to...": Frame boundaries in terms of your own actions rather than requirements for your partner's behavior. "I will leave the room when you start yelling" is more powerful than "I need you to stop yelling at me" because you control your own actions.

"This conversation is over" vs "Let's not talk about this now": Use definitive language rather than suggestions when ending harmful discussions. Personality disorders often involve pushing past social cues that would stop most people.

"I'm not available for that" vs "I can't do that right now": Avoid language that implies your boundaries are temporary or situational.

"I'm not available to manage your emotions about work stress" is clearer than "I can't help you with work stress today."

"That doesn't work for me" vs "That makes me feel bad": Focus on practical outcomes rather than emotional impacts when setting boundaries. Personality disorders often involve using your emotions against you or dismissing your feelings as invalid.

Scripts for Specific Situations:

When Your Partner Demands Explanations for Boundaries: "This is my decision and I'm not going to debate it." "I've told you my position on this and I'm not changing it." "You don't have to understand my boundary, but you do need to respect it."

When Your Partner Tests Your Boundaries: "I said no, and that hasn't changed." "I'm going to take a break from this conversation now." "This is exactly what I said I wouldn't do."

When Your Partner Tries to Make You Feel Guilty: "I understand you're disappointed, and this is still my decision." "Your feelings about my boundary don't change my boundary." "I can see you're upset, and I'm not going to change my mind."

Case Example 2: Finding Language That Actually Works David struggled with setting boundaries with his wife Sarah, who had dependent personality disorder, because his natural communication style involved extensive explanations and collaborative problem-solving. These approaches backfired with Sarah because they gave her opportunities to argue against his boundaries or to make his limits feel like negotiations rather than decisions.

David's initial boundary attempts sounded like: "Sarah, I think it would be better for both of us if you tried to make some decisions independently because I think it would help you build confidence and I'm feeling overwhelmed by making decisions for both of us all the time."

This approach invited Sarah to argue about David's assessment of her needs, question his feelings of being overwhelmed, and propose alternatives that would allow her to continue avoiding decision-making. The boundary became a lengthy discussion rather than a clear limit.

David learned to use more direct language: "I won't be available for decision-making calls during work hours." When Sarah asked why or tried to discuss exceptions, David would repeat: "I won't be available for decision-making calls during work hours." This approach removed the invitation for negotiation and made David's boundary clear and consistent.

Why Boundaries Feel Selfish But Aren't

The most common reason boundaries fail in personality disorder relationships is that partners feel selfish or cruel for setting limits when their loved one appears to be genuinely suffering. Your partner's distress about your boundaries feels like proof that you're being harsh or unloving, especially when their emotional reactions are intense and dramatic.

Understanding why boundaries trigger such strong reactions helps you maintain them despite the emotional pressure to give in.

Why Personality Disorders React Strongly to Boundaries:

Boundaries Threaten Control: Many personality disorders involve attempts to control their environment and relationships as a way of managing internal chaos. Your boundaries represent loss of control, which triggers anxiety and desperate attempts to regain influence over you.

Boundaries Challenge Schemas: If your partner operates from abandonment fears, your boundaries feel like evidence that you're preparing to leave. If they operate from entitlement beliefs, your boundaries feel like unfair restrictions on their deserved treatment.

Boundaries Require Internal Resources: Respecting your boundaries means your partner must develop their own coping skills rather than relying on you to manage their emotional needs. This feels overwhelming when they lack confidence in their ability to handle challenges independently.

Boundaries Expose the Dysfunction: When you stop accommodating disordered behaviors, those behaviors become more obvious to both of you. This can trigger shame and defensive reactions designed to make you return to your previous accommodating patterns.

Why Your Boundaries Are Actually Loving:

Boundaries Model Healthy Relationships: By maintaining limits, you show your partner what respectful relationships look like rather than enabling patterns that will damage future relationships.

Boundaries Encourage Growth: When you stop rescuing your partner from the consequences of their choices, they have opportunities to develop their own skills and confidence.

Boundaries Protect the Relationship: Relationships without boundaries often end in resentment and exhaustion. Maintaining limits preserves your ability to continue loving and supporting your partner within healthy parameters.

Boundaries Reduce Enabling: Accommodating disordered behaviors often makes those behaviors worse over time. Boundaries interrupt the cycle of escalating dysfunction.

Enforcing Consequences with Compassion

The hardest part of boundary-setting involves following through with consequences when your boundaries are violated. Your natural impulse might be to give warnings, make exceptions, or provide additional chances, but inconsistent enforcement teaches your partner that your boundaries aren't real.

Effective Consequence Strategies:

Natural Consequences: Allow situations to play out naturally rather than protecting your partner from the results of their choices. If they refuse to participate in social planning, they experience the consequences of missed events rather than you handling everything for them.

Logical Consequences: Create outcomes that directly relate to the boundary violation. If your partner violates your privacy by reading your texts, the consequence might be that you no longer leave your phone accessible rather than a punishment unrelated to the violation.

Consistent Application: Apply consequences every time boundaries are violated rather than making exceptions based on circumstances or your partner's emotional state. Consistency is more important than severity.

Compassionate Delivery: You can enforce consequences while still expressing care for your partner. "I can see you're really struggling right now, and I'm still not going to engage with you while you're calling me names."

Case Example 3: Learning to Follow Through Jennifer had set a boundary with her boyfriend Mark, who had obsessive-compulsive personality disorder, about his criticism of her housekeeping. Jennifer told Mark that she wouldn't stay in conversations where he was criticizing her cleaning methods or pointing out things she had done "wrong."

Initially, Jennifer would warn Mark when he started being critical, give him chances to change the subject, and only leave conversations after multiple violations of her boundary. This approach taught Mark that Jennifer's boundaries weren't serious and that he could continue his critical behavior as long as he was willing to endure some complaints from Jennifer.

Jennifer learned to enforce her boundary immediately and consistently. The first critical comment would result in Jennifer leaving the room without warnings or explanations. This was difficult because Mark would become distressed about Jennifer's departure and would promise to stop being critical if she would just stay and discuss the issue.

Jennifer had to learn that Mark's distress about consequences didn't mean the consequences were wrong. Mark's emotional reaction to Jennifer's boundary was exactly what the boundary was designed to address—his expectation that Jennifer would accommodate his critical behavior rather than protecting herself from it.

When Boundaries Become Walls: Finding Balance

While boundaries are essential for personality disorder relationships, they can sometimes become walls that prevent any real intimacy or connection. The challenge lies in maintaining protection for yourself while still allowing space for love, growth, and genuine partnership.

Signs Your Boundaries May Be Too Rigid:

Complete Emotional Shutdown: If you've become so protective that you can't be vulnerable or emotionally present with your partner, your boundaries may have become barriers to intimacy.

Punishment Rather Than Protection: If your boundaries feel like ways to punish your partner for their disorder rather than ways to protect your well-being, they may be serving the wrong purpose.

No Room for Growth: If your boundaries don't allow space for your partner to change and improve their behavior, they may be based on past experiences rather than current realities.

Relationship Stagnation: If boundaries have eliminated all risk and challenge from your relationship, they may also have eliminated opportunities for connection and growth.

Finding Healthy Balance:

Regular Boundary Review: Periodically assess whether your boundaries are still necessary and appropriate based on current relationship dynamics rather than past experiences.

Graduated Boundaries: Create different levels of boundaries based on your partner's current stability and behavior rather than applying maximum restrictions all the time.

Positive Boundaries: Include boundaries that create space for good things (time for fun, intimacy, growth) rather than only boundaries that prevent bad things.

Flexibility Within Limits: Allow some variation in how boundaries are applied while maintaining the core protective elements.

Your Personal Boundary Blueprint

Creating effective boundaries requires understanding your own needs, limits, and values rather than simply copying boundaries that work for other people. Your boundary blueprint should reflect your unique situation, personality, and goals for your relationship.

Creating Your Blueprint:

1. **Identify Your Non-Negotiables**: What behaviors or situations are absolutely unacceptable regardless of circumstances? These become your firmest boundaries.

2. **Assess Your Capacity**: What can you handle on good days versus difficult days? Create flexible boundaries that account for your varying energy and emotional resources.

3. **Clarify Your Values**: What kind of relationship do you want? What behaviors align with your values? Use this vision to guide boundary decisions.

4. **Consider Your Goals**: Are you trying to improve your current relationship, protect yourself while deciding about the future, or prepare for separation? Your goals should influence your boundary choices.

5. **Plan Your Implementation**: How will you communicate boundaries? What consequences will you enforce? How will you maintain consistency? Preparation increases success.

6. **Build Support Systems**: Who can help you maintain your boundaries when you feel tempted to give in? Having support makes boundary-setting more sustainable.

The Foundation of Self-Respect

Boundaries in personality disorder relationships aren't about changing your partner or punishing them for their condition. They're about creating conditions where you can maintain your well-being, self-respect, and capacity for love while dealing with challenging relationship dynamics.

Effective boundaries require courage to prioritize your own needs, wisdom to distinguish between your partner's genuine struggles and manipulative behaviors, and commitment to follow through even when doing so feels difficult or cruel.

The goal isn't to create perfect boundaries that solve all your relationship problems. The goal is to create sustainable limits that allow you to stay emotionally and physically healthy while making informed decisions about your relationship's future.

Your boundaries will change as you grow, as your partner changes (or doesn't), and as your relationship evolves. The skills you develop in setting and maintaining boundaries will serve you not just in your current relationship but in all future relationships and life challenges.

Key Insights for Boundary Setting

- Different personality disorders require different boundary approaches based on their unique manipulation patterns and triggers

- Effective boundary language is direct, non-negotiable, and doesn't invite argument or lengthy explanations

- Guilt about setting boundaries is normal but doesn't indicate that boundaries are wrong or harmful to your partner

- Consequences must be enforced consistently and immediately to establish that boundaries are real and will be maintained

- Boundaries can become walls that prevent intimacy if they're too rigid or punitive rather than protective

- Personal boundary blueprints should reflect your individual needs, values, and relationship goals rather than generic advice

Chapter 16: Staying vs. Leaving

- The Hardest Decision

The decision keeps you awake at 3 AM, cycling through the same impossible questions. Do you stay and continue trying to make love work with someone whose personality disorder creates constant challenges? Or do you leave and face the guilt of abandoning someone who can't help their mental health condition? Every conversation with friends and family seems to push you toward one choice or the other, but they don't live in your relationship. They don't understand the daily reality of loving someone whose brain works differently from most people's.

The Decision Matrix: Factors That Matter Most

Making the stay-or-leave decision requires moving beyond emotions and analyzing the concrete factors that determine if your relationship has a realistic chance of improvement or if continuing will only cause more damage to both partners. This isn't about giving up on love— it's about making informed choices based on evidence rather than hope alone.

Factors That Suggest Staying May Be Worth It:

Your Partner Acknowledges Their Disorder: They recognize that their behavior patterns are problematic and accept responsibility for their role in relationship difficulties rather than blaming everything on external circumstances or your reactions.

Active Treatment Engagement: They're consistently attending therapy, taking prescribed medications if appropriate, and genuinely working to develop better coping strategies rather than just going through the motions to appease you.

Measurable Progress Over Time: You can identify specific improvements in their behavior, emotional regulation, or communication skills over months or years, not just temporary changes during crisis periods.

Absence of Abuse: While personality disorder behaviors can be challenging and hurtful, the relationship doesn't involve physical violence, threats, financial exploitation, or systematic emotional abuse designed to control or destroy you.

Your Mental Health Remains Intact: You're able to maintain your own identity, relationships, goals, and emotional well-being while supporting your partner through their challenges.

Mutual Effort: Both of you are working to improve the relationship dynamics, learning new skills, and making changes rather than all the effort coming from one side.

Factors That Suggest Leaving May Be Necessary:

Complete Lack of Insight: Your partner sees no problems with their behavior and believes all relationship issues stem from your inadequacies, reactions, or mental health problems.

Treatment Resistance: They refuse professional help, discontinue treatment when symptoms improve, or attend therapy only to prove they're right rather than to make changes.

Escalating Dysfunction: The relationship patterns are getting worse over time rather than staying stable or improving, with increased frequency or intensity of problematic behaviors.

Presence of Abuse: Any form of physical violence, threats, financial exploitation, or systematic emotional abuse that's designed to control your behavior or destroy your sense of reality.

Your Deteriorating Health: You're developing anxiety, depression, trauma symptoms, or physical health problems from the chronic stress of the relationship dynamics.

Impact on Children: If you have children, their emotional or physical well-being is being compromised by the personality disorder dynamics in your home.

Red Flags You Can't Ignore

According to research from Mylifereflections and FHE Health, certain behaviors in personality disorder relationships represent serious safety risks that require immediate attention rather than long-term relationship work. These red flags indicate that your physical or psychological safety is in immediate danger and that leaving may be necessary for survival.

Physical Safety Red Flags:

Escalating Violence: Any progression from verbal threats to physical intimidation to actual violence, regardless of apologies or promises that it won't happen again.

Threats of Harm: Direct or indirect threats to hurt you, themselves, children, pets, or other people important to you, especially when combined with access to weapons or history of violence.

Property Destruction: Breaking your belongings, punching walls, or other displays of physical aggression that serve as warnings about what could happen to you.

Isolation Tactics: Preventing you from working, seeing friends or family, or having access to transportation or communication as ways of controlling your ability to leave or get help.

Financial Control: Taking control of all money, hiding assets, preventing you from working, or creating financial dependence that makes leaving practically impossible.

Psychological Safety Red Flags:

Systematic Gaslighting: Deliberately distorting your reality, denying events you witnessed, or convincing you that your perceptions and memories are unreliable to the point where you question your own sanity.

Identity Destruction: Systematically attacking your self-worth, capabilities, and identity until you believe you're worthless and incapable of surviving without them.

Exploitation of Vulnerabilities: Using your mental health struggles, past trauma, or personal insecurities as weapons against you or as reasons why you deserve poor treatment.

Suicide Threats for Control: Using threats of self-harm as tools to manipulate your behavior, prevent you from leaving, or force you to provide attention and care.

Case Example 1: Recognizing When Love Isn't Enough Rebecca spent four years trying to make her marriage work with David, who had narcissistic personality disorder. Rebecca loved David and could see moments of the person he could be when he wasn't consumed by his need for control and admiration. She kept hoping that with enough patience, therapy, and understanding, David would develop empathy and learn to treat her with respect.

Over the four years, Rebecca documented her attempts to improve their relationship. She attended individual therapy to learn better communication skills, couple's therapy where David used the sessions to prove Rebecca was the problem, and support groups where she learned about narcissistic abuse. Rebecca modified her behavior, adjusted her expectations, and tried multiple approaches to help David understand how his behavior affected her.

During this time, David's behavior actually worsened rather than improved. He became more controlling, more critical, and more convinced that Rebecca's complaints about his behavior were evidence of her mental instability. David used information from therapy sessions to refine his manipulation tactics and began involving Rebecca's family and friends in campaigns to prove that Rebecca was the real problem in their marriage.

The turning point came when Rebecca realized that her love and effort couldn't create empathy in someone who lacked the capacity for genuine concern about others. David's narcissistic personality disorder meant that he experienced Rebecca's pain as inconvenience rather than as something worthy of compassion or behavior change.

Rebecca made the difficult decision to leave when she accepted that David's lack of empathy wasn't something she could fix through better communication, more understanding, or greater patience. The problem wasn't their relationship dynamics—it was David's fundamental inability to care about anyone's needs except his own.

Financial Planning for Potential Separation

Leaving personality disorder relationships often involves additional financial complexity because these relationships frequently involve financial manipulation, control, or exploitation. Planning for potential separation requires protecting yourself financially while maintaining the resources necessary to leave safely if needed.

Financial Protection Strategies:

Document Your Assets: Keep records of all bank accounts, retirement funds, property, investments, and other assets that belong to you or that you contributed to during the relationship.

Secure Independent Access: Maintain at least one bank account that your partner cannot access and ensure you have independent access to some funds for emergencies.

Credit Monitoring: Check your credit reports regularly for accounts opened in your name without your permission, which is common in abusive personality disorder relationships.

Important Documents: Keep copies of identification, financial records, insurance policies, and other important documents in a secure location your partner cannot access.

Legal Consultation: Meet with a family law attorney to understand your rights and options before making final decisions about leaving, especially if you're married or have significant shared assets.

Employment Protection: If your partner has interfered with your ability to work or has damaged your professional reputation, document these incidents and consider whether you need to rebuild your career independence.

Case Example 2: Financial Recovery After Leaving Maria discovered after leaving her husband Jake that he had been systematically destroying her financial independence for years. Jake had convinced Maria to quit her job to focus on their relationship, had opened credit cards in her name without her knowledge, and had used her excellent credit to secure loans that he spent on his own interests.

When Maria decided to leave, she realized that Jake had created financial dependence that made separation practically difficult. Maria had no current income, damaged credit from Jake's financial abuse, and no independent housing or transportation options.

Maria worked with a domestic violence financial advocate to develop a plan for financial recovery. Maria secured temporary housing through a friend, obtained copies of all financial records, and began the process of disputing fraudulent accounts Jake had opened in her name.

Maria also had to rebuild her career after years away from the workforce. Maria started with part-time work in her previous field and gradually rebuilt her professional reputation and financial independence. The process took nearly two years, but Maria was able to achieve financial stability and independence.

Most importantly, Maria learned to recognize financial abuse red flags that would prevent her from falling into similar situations in future relationships. Maria's experience taught her that financial independence isn't just practical—it's essential for safety in relationships with personality disorder dynamics.

Protecting Children: When Their Wellbeing Comes First

According to research from Grouport and PubMed Central, children in households with personality disorder dynamics are at risk for developing their own mental health issues, learning unhealthy relationship patterns, and experiencing trauma that affects their development. Protecting children often becomes the deciding factor in stay-or-leave decisions.

How Personality Disorders Affect Children:

Emotional Dysregulation Modeling: Children learn that emotional intensity, manipulation, and chaos are normal parts of relationships rather than learning healthy emotional regulation skills.

Parentification: Children may be forced to manage the personality disordered parent's emotions, serve as confidants for adult problems, or take responsibility for household stability.

Triangulation: Children get pulled into adult conflicts, used as messengers between parents, or forced to choose sides in parental disputes.

Inconsistent Parenting: The personality disordered parent may alternate between over-involvement and neglect, creating attachment insecurity in children.

Reality Distortion: Children may learn they can't trust their own perceptions because the personality disordered parent constantly rewrites reality to serve their own needs.

Protection Strategies for Children:

Validate Their Reality: When the personality disordered parent gaslights or manipulates children, provide gentle reality checks that help them trust their own perceptions.

Emotional Education: Teach children about healthy emotional regulation, appropriate boundaries, and normal relationship dynamics to counter what they observe at home.

Professional Support: Consider therapy for children who are showing signs of anxiety, depression, behavioral problems, or developmental delays related to the household dynamics.

Safety Planning: If the personality disordered parent's behavior is escalating or becoming dangerous, develop safety plans that protect children from potential harm.

Documentation: Keep records of concerning incidents involving the children, as this information may be crucial for custody decisions or legal protection.

Case Example 3: Choosing Children's Safety Over Relationship Preservation Jennifer stayed in her marriage to Mark, who had borderline personality disorder, for three additional years because she hoped their family could remain intact if she just learned to manage his emotional dysregulation better. Jennifer focused on protecting their two young children from Mark's emotional outbursts while trying to help Mark develop better coping skills.

Over time, Jennifer realized that her children were being damaged despite her efforts to protect them. Her older child had developed anxiety and perfectionist tendencies, constantly monitoring Mark's moods and trying to prevent his emotional meltdowns. Her younger child had become withdrawn and was showing developmental delays that Jennifer's pediatrician attributed to chronic stress.

The turning point came when Jennifer's older child told her that they felt responsible for Mark's happiness and were scared to express their own needs or feelings because they might upset him. Jennifer realized that by staying in the marriage, she was teaching her children that their emotional needs were less important than managing other people's mental health.

Jennifer made the difficult decision to separate from Mark when she accepted that her children's developmental needs were more important than her desire to keep their family intact. Jennifer worked with a family therapist to help her children understand that Mark's behavior wasn't their fault and that they deserved relationships where their feelings mattered.

The separation was traumatic for everyone involved, but within six months, Jennifer noticed improvements in both children's anxiety levels and emotional expression. Her children began showing more confidence, creativity, and willingness to express their own needs and feelings rather than constantly focusing on managing adult emotions.

The "One More Try" Trap

Many partners in personality disorder relationships get stuck in cycles of "one more try"—giving their relationship another chance after each crisis, promise to change, or brief period of improvement. This pattern can continue for years or decades, preventing you from making clear decisions about your future while keeping you trapped in cycles of hope and disappointment.

Why the "One More Try" Pattern Develops:

Intermittent Reinforcement: Personality disorder relationships often involve periods of intense connection and love mixed with periods of dysfunction. This creates an addiction-like pattern where you keep trying to recapture the good times.

Trauma Bonding: The cycle of abuse followed by reconciliation creates strong psychological bonds that feel like love but are actually trauma responses that make leaving feel impossible.

Sunk Cost Fallacy: After investing years in a relationship, leaving feels like admitting that all your time, effort, and love were wasted rather than recognizing that some situations can't be fixed regardless of investment.

Hope Addiction: The personality disordered partner's promises to change and brief periods of improvement create hope that keeps you engaged even when evidence suggests that lasting change isn't occurring.

Breaking the "One More Try" Cycle:

Set Clear Criteria for Change: Instead of hoping for improvement, define specific, measurable changes you need to see within specific timeframes.

Track Patterns Over Time: Keep records of promises made, improvements claimed, and actual behavior changes to see patterns rather than focusing on isolated incidents.

External Reality Checks: Work with therapists, support groups, or trusted friends who can provide objective perspectives on whether real change is occurring.

Focus on Trajectory: Assess whether the overall direction of your relationship is improving, staying the same, or getting worse rather than focusing on temporary fluctuations.

Making Peace with Your Decision

The hardest part of the stay-or-leave decision often isn't making the choice—it's living with the choice afterward. Both staying and leaving involve losses and difficulties that require grieving and acceptance.

Making Peace with Staying:

Accept the Limitations: If you choose to stay, accept that some aspects of your relationship will always be challenging and may never match your ideal vision of partnership.

Focus on What You Can Control: Direct your energy toward your own growth, coping skills, and well-being rather than trying to change your partner or fix your relationship.

Build External Support: Maintain friendships, hobbies, and interests that provide fulfillment outside your relationship so that your entire happiness doesn't depend on your partner's mental health.

Regular Reassessment: Periodically evaluate whether staying continues to make sense based on current circumstances rather than past investment or future hopes.

Making Peace with Leaving:

Grieve the Relationship You Hoped For: Allow yourself to mourn not just the actual relationship but the relationship you thought you could create with enough love and effort.

Release Responsibility for Their Future: Accept that leaving doesn't make you responsible for what happens to your partner afterward, just as staying wouldn't guarantee their well-being.

Focus on Your Growth: Use the experience as information about your own needs, boundaries, and relationship goals rather than viewing it as failure or wasted time.

Build New Foundations: Create new routines, relationships, and life structures that support the person you want to become rather than the person you were in your previous relationship.

The Courage of Honest Assessment

The stay-or-leave decision ultimately requires brutally honest assessment of your relationship's reality rather than its potential. This means looking at evidence rather than promises, patterns rather than exceptions, and trajectory rather than hope.

Neither choice is inherently right or wrong. Some personality disorder relationships can become satisfying and stable with appropriate treatment, boundaries, and realistic expectations. Others represent fundamental incompatibilities that no amount of love or effort can overcome.

Your decision should be based on your actual experience rather than societal expectations, your own needs rather than your partner's preferences, and realistic assessment rather than wishful thinking. The courage to make difficult decisions—and to live with their consequences—represents one of the most important skills you can develop.

The goal isn't to make the perfect decision but to make an informed decision that honors your values, protects your well-being, and creates the best possible outcomes given your specific circumstances and constraints.

Key Insights for Decision Making

- The stay-or-leave decision should be based on measurable evidence of change and improvement rather than hope and potential

- Safety assessment is crucial because certain personality disorder behaviors represent immediate physical or psychological dangers

- Financial planning protects your ability to leave safely and rebuild your life if separation becomes necessary

- Children's wellbeing often becomes the deciding factor because personality disorder dynamics can cause lasting developmental damage

- The "one more try" pattern can trap partners in cycles of hope and disappointment that prevent clear decision-making

- Making peace with your decision requires accepting losses and focusing on what you can control regardless of your choice

Chapter 17: Healing and Moving Forward

The relationship is over, but the confusion remains. You find yourself questioning every memory, wondering if things were as bad as they seemed, and struggling to trust your own perceptions about what constitutes normal treatment in relationships. Friends tell you to "move on" and "focus on the positive," but they don't understand that personality disorder relationships leave invisible scars that affect your ability to recognize healthy connections and trust your own judgment about people and situations.

Trauma Recovery for Partners: You're Not Crazy

According to research from Choosing Therapy and related mental health sources, partners in personality disorder relationships often develop trauma symptoms similar to post-traumatic stress disorder, but their trauma isn't recognized or validated because it doesn't fit the typical narrative of abuse. Your trauma is real, even if it doesn't look like what most people imagine when they think of relationship abuse.

Common Trauma Symptoms in Partners:

Hypervigilance: You constantly monitor other people's moods and reactions, looking for signs of disapproval, anger, or rejection because you learned that missing these cues could lead to emotional explosions or punishment.

Emotional Numbing: After years of having your emotions invalidated, criticized, or used against you, you may have learned to disconnect from your own feelings as a protective mechanism.

Memory Distortion: Gaslighting and reality distortion may have affected your confidence in your own memories and perceptions, making you question what really happened in various situations.

Relationship Anxiety: You may feel anxious about normal relationship interactions, constantly worrying that you've done something wrong or that your partner is losing interest based on minor changes in their behavior.

Identity Confusion: After years of being criticized, controlled, or told that your perceptions are wrong, you may struggle to know who you are or what you actually want and need.

Somatic Symptoms: Chronic stress from personality disorder relationships often manifests in physical symptoms like headaches, stomach problems, sleep disturbances, or other stress-related health issues.

Why Your Trauma Response Makes Sense:

Chronic Stress Activation: Personality disorder relationships involve unpredictable emotional intensity that keeps your nervous system in constant alert mode, leading to physical and emotional exhaustion.

Reality Distortion: When someone consistently tells you that your perceptions are wrong, your brain's ability to process and trust information becomes compromised, creating confusion and self-doubt.

Attachment Trauma: The push-pull dynamics common in personality disorder relationships create insecure attachment patterns that affect your ability to feel safe in future relationships.

Complex Grief: You're grieving not just the relationship but also your sense of reality, your confidence in your judgment, and your belief in your ability to recognize healthy relationships.

Case Example 1: Sarah's Recovery Journey Sarah left her five-year relationship with Marcus, who had narcissistic personality disorder, but found that ending the relationship didn't immediately resolve her emotional difficulties. Sarah experienced panic attacks when people disagreed with her opinions, constantly apologized for normal behaviors, and found herself unable to make simple decisions without seeking extensive input from others.

Sarah initially tried to move on quickly, dating new people and focusing on building a new life. But Sarah's trauma symptoms interfered with her ability to form healthy new relationships. Sarah would become anxious when dates didn't respond to texts immediately, would misinterpret normal relationship conflicts as signs of impending abandonment, and would find herself attracted to people who displayed some of the same controlling behaviors that Marcus had shown.

Sarah realized she needed professional help to address the trauma from her relationship with Marcus before she could build healthy new relationships. Sarah worked with a therapist who specialized in narcissistic abuse recovery and learned that her symptoms were normal responses to abnormal treatment rather than signs of mental illness.

Sarah's recovery involved learning to trust her own perceptions again, developing confidence in her ability to recognize red flags in relationships, and rebuilding her sense of identity separate from her role as Marcus's partner. This process took nearly two years, but Sarah eventually developed the skills and confidence to form healthy relationships based on mutual respect rather than trauma bonding.

Rebuilding Your Identity After the Relationship

Personality disorder relationships often involve gradual erosion of your individual identity as you adapt your behavior, interests, and self-expression to accommodate your partner's needs and avoid triggering their symptoms. Recovery requires rediscovering who you are when you're not managing someone else's emotional state or walking on eggshells to prevent conflicts.

Identity Recovery Process:

Reconnect with Pre-Relationship Interests: What activities, hobbies, or interests did you enjoy before your relationship began? These often provide clues about your authentic self that got submerged during the relationship.

Explore Suppressed Aspects: What parts of your personality did you learn to hide or minimize during your relationship? Recovery often involves giving yourself permission to express traits that your partner criticized or discouraged.

Rebuild Social Connections: Reconnect with friends and family members you may have lost touch with during your relationship, and work on developing new friendships based on your authentic interests and values.

Rediscover Your Preferences: You may have become so focused on your partner's preferences that you've forgotten your own. Spend time exploring what you actually like and want rather than what you think you should like.

Develop Independent Goals: What do you want to achieve in your life independent of romantic relationships? Career goals, personal growth objectives, creative projects, or other aspirations that belong entirely to you.

Practice Self-Advocacy: Learn to express your needs, opinions, and preferences in low-risk situations to rebuild confidence in your right to have and express your own thoughts and feelings.

Case Example 2: Rediscovering Mark's Authentic Self Mark realized during his recovery from his relationship with Jessica, who had borderline personality disorder, that he had completely lost touch with his own interests and preferences. During their three-year relationship, Mark had focused entirely on managing Jessica's emotional crises and had gradually abandoned all activities that didn't directly relate to their relationship.

Mark couldn't remember what he enjoyed doing in his free time, what types of music or movies he preferred, or even what foods he liked to eat because he had made all these decisions based on Jessica's preferences and emotional needs. Mark had become so skilled at reading Jessica's moods and anticipating her needs that he had lost the ability to recognize his own feelings and desires.

Mark's recovery began with very basic self-discovery exercises. Mark spent time in bookstores noticing which books attracted his attention, listened to different types of music to see what resonated with him, and tried various activities to rediscover what brought him joy and satisfaction.

Mark was surprised to discover interests he hadn't realized he had—photography, hiking, and cooking—that had been completely absent from his relationship with Jessica because they didn't fit with her lifestyle or interests. Mark also reconnected with friends he had lost touch with and discovered that he enjoyed quieter, more thoughtful social interactions than the dramatic, crisis-focused social life he had shared with Jessica.

Most importantly, Mark learned to make decisions based on his own preferences rather than trying to anticipate other people's reactions. This skill became essential for building healthier relationships where he could be authentic rather than constantly adapting to avoid conflict or emotional explosions.

Dating Again: Recognizing Patterns and Red Flags

One of the most challenging aspects of recovery involves learning to recognize healthy relationship patterns versus the dysfunction you became accustomed to during your personality disorder relationship. Many survivors find themselves attracted to familiar patterns that feel like "chemistry" but are actually trauma responses to unhealthy dynamics.

Common Dating Challenges for Survivors:

Attraction to Familiar Dysfunction: The intensity and drama of personality disorder relationships can make healthy relationships feel boring or emotionally flat by comparison.

Missing Red Flags: You may have become so accustomed to managing difficult behaviors that you normalize warning signs that should prompt concern.

Overreacting to Normal Conflict: Healthy relationships involve disagreements and conflicts, but these may trigger anxiety responses if you're accustomed to conflicts that escalate into emotional warfare.

Trust Issues: You may find it difficult to trust new partners or may swing between excessive trust (trying to prove you're not paranoid) and excessive suspicion (trying to protect yourself from future harm).

People-Pleasing Patterns: You may automatically adapt your behavior to avoid conflict or displeasure, preventing partners from getting to know your authentic self.

Red Flags to Watch For:

Love Bombing: Excessive attention, gifts, declarations of love, or future planning very early in relationships often indicate manipulation rather than genuine connection.

Boundary Testing: Partners who push against your limits, make exceptions to your boundaries, or argue with your "no" responses are showing disrespect that will likely escalate.

Gaslighting Behaviors: Anyone who tells you that your memories are wrong, your feelings are invalid, or your perceptions are unrealistic is engaging in psychological manipulation.

Control Tactics: Partners who want to monitor your communications, control your schedule, or isolate you from friends and family are displaying possessive behaviors that will worsen over time.

Emotional Manipulation: Using guilt, threats, or emotional explosions to influence your behavior indicates someone who lacks healthy communication skills and emotional regulation.

Case Example 3: Learning to Recognize Healthy vs Unhealthy Attraction Lisa found herself repeatedly attracted to men who displayed subtle signs of narcissistic or controlling behavior during her first year of dating after leaving her marriage to David. Lisa would feel intense chemistry with men who were charming, confident, and seemed to have strong opinions about everything, but these relationships would quickly become one-sided with Lisa adapting her behavior to maintain her partner's interest and approval.

Lisa worked with her therapist to understand why she felt drawn to these familiar patterns and how to recognize the difference between healthy confidence and narcissistic entitlement. Lisa learned that healthy partners would show interest in her opinions, respect her boundaries, and demonstrate empathy when she expressed concerns or needs.

Lisa also learned to pay attention to how she felt in different relationships. With unhealthy partners, Lisa felt anxious, constantly worried about doing something wrong, and focused on earning approval. With healthy partners, Lisa felt more relaxed, able to be authentic, and confident that minor conflicts wouldn't threaten the relationship.

Most importantly, Lisa learned to take relationships slowly and observe patterns over time rather than making decisions based on initial chemistry or attraction. Lisa discovered that healthy relationships often felt less intense initially but provided much greater satisfaction and security over time than the dramatic ups and downs she had experienced in dysfunctional relationships.

Post-Traumatic Growth: Finding Meaning in the Pain

While personality disorder relationships cause genuine trauma and suffering, many survivors eventually experience post-traumatic growth—positive psychological changes that result from struggling with highly challenging circumstances. This doesn't mean the trauma was worth it or that you should be grateful for the experience, but it recognizes that humans often develop strength and wisdom through surviving difficult situations.

Areas of Post-Traumatic Growth:

Increased Empathy and Compassion: Surviving psychological manipulation and emotional abuse often increases your ability to recognize and respond to others' suffering with genuine understanding.

Stronger Boundaries: Learning to protect yourself from personality disorder manipulation often results in better boundary-setting skills that improve all your relationships.

Greater Self-Knowledge: The process of recovering your identity and healing from trauma often leads to deeper understanding of your values, needs, and goals than you had before the challenging relationship.

Improved Discernment: Learning to recognize manipulation, gaslighting, and other unhealthy behaviors makes you better at identifying trustworthy people and healthy relationship dynamics.

Resilience and Coping Skills: Surviving personality disorder relationships often develops emotional resilience and coping abilities that help you handle future challenges with greater confidence.

Spiritual or Philosophical Growth: Many survivors develop deeper spiritual practices or philosophical frameworks that provide meaning and perspective on their experiences.

Finding Meaning in Your Experience:

Helping Others: Many survivors find purpose in supporting other people who are dealing with similar relationship challenges through support groups, writing, or advocacy work.

Professional Development: Some survivors pursue careers in mental health, domestic violence advocacy, or other fields where their experience provides valuable insight and motivation.

Creative Expression: Writing, art, music, or other creative outlets can help process trauma while creating something meaningful from painful experiences.

Personal Growth: Using your experience as motivation for therapy, self-development, or spiritual practice can transform pain into wisdom and strength.

Success Stories: Partners Who Found Happiness

Recovery from personality disorder relationships is possible, and many survivors go on to build satisfying lives and healthy relationships. These success stories don't minimize the trauma or difficulty of the experience, but they provide hope and practical examples of what recovery can look like.

Types of Success Stories:

Building Healthy New Relationships: Many survivors eventually find partners who treat them with respect, empathy, and genuine care, creating relationships based on mutual support rather than drama and control.

Thriving as Single People: Some survivors discover that they prefer single life after years of managing someone else's emotional needs, finding fulfillment in careers, friendships, hobbies, and personal growth.

Successful Co-Parenting: Parents who share children with personality disordered ex-partners often learn to create stable, protective environments for their children while maintaining necessary boundaries with their co-parent.

Professional Achievement: Many survivors redirect the energy they once spent managing dysfunctional relationships into career success, creative projects, or community involvement that brings satisfaction and recognition.

Helping Others Heal: Some survivors become therapists, support group leaders, writers, or advocates who use their experience to help other people navigate similar challenges.

Your Next Chapter Starts Now

Recovery from personality disorder relationships isn't about returning to who you were before the relationship began—it's about becoming someone new who incorporates the wisdom gained from surviving challenging circumstances. This process takes time, often requires professional support, and involves both grief for what was lost and hope for what's possible in your future.

Your next chapter may look different than you originally imagined, but it can be built on a foundation of self-respect, healthy boundaries, and genuine understanding of what you need and deserve in relationships. The skills you develop during recovery— emotional regulation, boundary setting, reality testing, and self-advocacy—will serve you not just in romantic relationships but in all areas of your life.

The goal isn't to forget your experience or pretend it didn't affect you. The goal is to integrate your experience in ways that make you stronger, wiser, and more capable of creating the life you want to live.

The Phoenix Rises

Recovery from personality disorder relationships represents one of the most challenging psychological journeys you can undertake. It requires rebuilding your sense of reality, rediscovering your authentic self, and learning to trust your judgment again after having it systematically undermined.

The process isn't linear—you'll have good days and setbacks, moments of clarity and periods of confusion. But each step forward, each boundary maintained, each red flag recognized, each healthy choice made, contributes to your growing strength and wisdom.

Your experience with personality disorder relationships, while painful, has taught you things about human psychology, relationship dynamics, and your own resilience that many people never learn. This knowledge, combined with appropriate healing and growth work, can become the foundation for a life of greater authenticity, stronger relationships, and deeper self-respect than you might have achieved otherwise.

The person you become through this healing process—someone who understands manipulation but chooses authenticity, who has experienced betrayal but chooses trust wisely, who has been diminished but chooses self-respect—is someone worth becoming, regardless of how difficult the journey has been.

Key Insights for Recovery and Growth

- Trauma symptoms after personality disorder relationships are normal responses to abnormal treatment and require professional support for full healing

- Identity recovery involves rediscovering interests, preferences, and aspects of self that were suppressed during the dysfunctional relationship

- Dating again requires learning to distinguish between healthy attraction and trauma bonding to familiar dysfunction patterns

- Post-traumatic growth can result from surviving personality disorder relationships, leading to increased empathy, better boundaries, and greater resilience

- Success stories take many forms, from healthy new relationships to thriving single life to helping others heal from similar experiences

- Recovery is about becoming someone new who integrates wisdom from difficult experiences rather than returning to who you were before

Chapter 18: Resources for the Journey

Your healing journey doesn't end with understanding personality disorders or making decisions about your relationship. Real recovery requires ongoing support, practical tools, and access to resources that can help you navigate the complex process of rebuilding your life. The challenge isn't finding resources—it's finding the right resources that understand the unique challenges of personality disorder relationships and provide practical help rather than generic advice.

Emergency Contacts and Crisis Resources

Personality disorder relationships can escalate into crisis situations that require immediate professional intervention. Having emergency resources readily available can mean the difference between managing a crisis effectively and finding yourself in a dangerous situation without adequate support.

National Crisis Resources:

National Suicide Prevention Lifeline: 988 - Available 24/7 for anyone experiencing suicidal thoughts or emotional distress, including partners dealing with threats or concerns about their loved one's safety.

National Domestic Violence Hotline: 1-800-799-7233 - Provides crisis intervention, safety planning, and referrals for people experiencing domestic abuse, including emotional and psychological abuse common in personality disorder relationships.

Crisis Text Line: Text HOME to 741741 - Free, confidential support via text message for anyone in crisis, available 24/7 with trained crisis counselors.

National Alliance on Mental Illness (NAMI) Helpline: 1-800-950-6264 - Provides information, referrals, and support for people affected by mental illness, including family members and partners of people with personality disorders.

SAMHSA National Helpline: 1-800-662-4357 - Substance Abuse and Mental Health Services Administration's treatment referral and information service for individuals and families facing mental health or substance use disorders.

Local Resources to Identify:

Regional Crisis Centers: Most areas have local crisis intervention centers that provide immediate support, safety planning, and connections to ongoing services.

Law Enforcement Mental Health Units: Many police departments have specialized units trained to respond to mental health crises with appropriate de-escalation techniques.

Hospital Emergency Departments: Know which local hospitals have psychiatric emergency services and 24-hour mental health professionals available.

Mobile Crisis Teams: Some areas have mobile mental health teams that can respond to crisis situations in homes or community settings.

When to Use Emergency Resources:

Immediate Safety Threats: Any situation involving threats of violence, actual violence, or credible concerns about physical safety for yourself, your partner, children, or others.

Suicide Threats or Attempts: When your partner threatens suicide, shows signs of planning self-harm, or attempts to hurt themselves, especially if these threats are used to control your behavior.

Severe Mental Health Crisis: When your partner experiences psychotic symptoms, complete emotional breakdown, or other severe mental health symptoms that require professional intervention.

Your Own Safety Concerns: When you feel unsafe, overwhelmed, or unable to cope with a crisis situation and need immediate support or guidance.

Recommended Books for Specific Disorders

Different personality disorders require different approaches and understanding. While this guide provides broad coverage, specialized books can offer deeper insight into specific conditions and their relationship impacts.

Borderline Personality Disorder:

- "Stop Walking on Eggshells" by Paul Mason and Randi Kreger - The classic guide for family members and partners, focusing on practical communication strategies and boundary setting.

- "Loving Someone with Borderline Personality Disorder" by Shari Manning - Written by a DBT expert, provides evidence-based strategies for maintaining relationships while protecting your own well-being.

Narcissistic Personality Disorder:

- "Will I Ever Be Good Enough?" by Karyl McBride - Focuses on recovery from narcissistic abuse and rebuilding self-worth after these relationships.

- "The Covert Passive-Aggressive Narcissist" by Debbie Mirza - Addresses the subtle forms of narcissistic abuse that are often difficult to identify and validate.

Avoidant Personality Disorder:

- "Attached" by Amir Levine and Rachel Heller - Explains attachment theory and how different attachment styles affect relationships, particularly relevant for avoidant patterns.

- "The Highly Sensitive Person" by Elaine Aron - While not specifically about personality disorders, provides helpful insights for understanding and supporting partners with extreme sensitivity to rejection.

Dependent Personality Disorder:

- "Codependent No More" by Melody Beattie - Classic resource for understanding and breaking codependent relationship patterns.

- "The New Codependency" by Melody Beattie - Updated approaches to creating healthy interdependence rather than unhealthy dependency.

Obsessive-Compulsive Personality Disorder:

- "Too Perfect" by Allan Mallinger and Jeannette DeWyze - Addresses perfectionism and rigid thinking patterns that characterize OCPD.

- "When Perfect Isn't Good Enough" by Martin Antony and Richard Swinson - Practical strategies for dealing with perfectionist tendencies in yourself and others.

Online Communities Worth Joining

Online support can provide connection, validation, and practical advice from people who understand your experience firsthand. However, not all online communities are helpful—some can become echo chambers or provide dangerous advice.

Recommended Online Communities:

BPDFamily.com: Well-moderated forum specifically for family members and partners of people with borderline personality disorder. Provides evidence-based information and peer support from experienced members.

Out of the FOG Forums: Comprehensive support community for people dealing with personality disorders in relationships. Covers all personality disorders with separate sections for different situations (dating, marriage, divorce, family).

Narcissistic Abuse Recovery Forums: Multiple platforms including Reddit communities like r/NarcissisticAbuse and dedicated websites that focus on healing from narcissistic relationships.

Psychology Today Support Groups: Online directory of virtual support groups led by mental health professionals, searchable by location and specialty.

NAMI Support Groups: National Alliance on Mental Illness offers both in-person and online support groups for family members and partners of people with mental health conditions.

7 Cups: Free emotional support platform where you can chat with trained listeners who understand relationship trauma and mental health challenges.

What to Look for in Online Communities:

Professional Moderation: Communities with mental health professionals or trained moderators who ensure discussions remain helpful and prevent harmful advice.

Evidence-Based Information: Groups that provide accurate information about personality disorders rather than speculation or stigmatizing content.

Recovery Focus: Communities that emphasize healing and growth rather than just venting or sharing trauma stories.

Respectful Boundaries: Groups that maintain respect for both partners and people with personality disorders, avoiding dehumanizing language or encouraging revenge.

What to Avoid Online:

Unmoderated Forums: Spaces where anyone can give advice without oversight, potentially including dangerous recommendations about leaving relationships or handling crises.

Diagnosis Communities: Groups focused on diagnosing partners rather than understanding and coping with behaviors.

Revenge-Focused Communities: Forums that encourage harmful actions toward partners with personality disorders or that demonize mental health conditions.

Commercial Sites: Platforms that primarily exist to sell products or services rather than provide genuine support.

Apps and Tools for Emotional Regulation

Technology can provide valuable support for managing the emotional challenges of personality disorder relationships and recovery. These tools can help you track patterns, practice coping skills, and maintain emotional balance during difficult times.

Mood and Pattern Tracking Apps:

Daylio: Simple mood tracking app that helps you identify patterns in your emotional responses to relationship events. Useful for recognizing triggers and tracking progress over time.

eMoods: More detailed mood tracking designed for people with mood disorders, but helpful for anyone who needs to monitor emotional patterns and stability.

MindShift: Anxiety management app that includes tools for challenging anxious thoughts and developing coping strategies for stress.

Sanvello: Comprehensive mental health app with mood tracking, anxiety management tools, and guided meditations specifically designed for relationship stress.

Crisis and Safety Apps:

My3: Personal safety app that allows you to designate three trusted contacts for crisis situations and provides quick access to professional crisis resources.

Safety Net: Domestic violence safety app that looks like a regular news app but provides access to safety planning tools and emergency contacts.

PTSD Coach: Developed by the VA, provides tools for managing trauma symptoms including grounding techniques and emotional regulation strategies.

Mindfulness and Emotional Regulation Apps:

Headspace: Guided meditation app with specific programs for relationships, stress, and emotional regulation.

Insight Timer: Free meditation app with thousands of guided meditations, including sessions specifically for relationship challenges and trauma recovery.

DBT Coach: App based on Dialectical Behavior Therapy principles, providing quick access to distress tolerance and emotional regulation skills.

Ten Percent Happier: Meditation app with programs specifically designed for people dealing with difficult relationships and emotional challenges.

Communication and Boundary Apps:

OurFamilyWizard: Co-parenting communication app that creates documented records of all interactions, useful for maintaining boundaries with personality disordered ex-partners.

Talking Parents: Another co-parenting app that provides neutral communication tools and documentation features.

Relationship Hero: Platform connecting users with relationship coaches for personalized advice about specific relationship challenges.

Legal Resources and Advocacy Groups

Personality disorder relationships often involve legal complications related to domestic violence, custody issues, financial abuse, or restraining orders. Knowing your legal options and having access to appropriate advocacy can be crucial for your safety and future security.

Legal Aid Organizations:

Legal Aid Society: Provides free or low-cost legal services for people who cannot afford private attorneys, including family law, domestic violence, and housing issues.

Domestic Violence Legal Clinics: Many areas have specialized legal clinics that provide free consultation and representation for domestic violence survivors.

Women's Law: National website providing legal information and resources specifically for women dealing with domestic violence and family law issues.

American Bar Association Pro Bono Programs: Connects people with volunteer attorneys who provide free legal services for qualifying cases.

Advocacy and Support Organizations:

National Coalition Against Domestic Violence: Provides resources, advocacy, and support for domestic violence survivors, including those experiencing emotional and psychological abuse.

Futures Without Violence: National organization focused on ending domestic and sexual violence through policy advocacy and education.

Local Domestic Violence Centers: Most communities have local organizations that provide legal advocacy, safety planning, and support services for abuse survivors.

Family Violence Prevention Centers: Often provide legal advocacy specifically for family law issues including divorce, custody, and restraining orders.

When You Need Legal Help:

Restraining Orders: If your partner has threatened violence, engaged in stalking, or created fear for your safety or your children's safety.

Custody Issues: When children are involved and you have concerns about their safety or well-being in your partner's care.

Financial Abuse: If your partner has stolen money, used your identity fraudulently, or hidden assets that belong to you.

Divorce Proceedings: Personality disorder relationships often involve high-conflict divorces that require specialized legal strategies.

Property Protection: When you need to secure important documents, assets, or belongings before leaving a relationship.

Creating Your Personal Support Team

Recovery from personality disorder relationships requires multiple types of support. Building a comprehensive support team provides you with different resources for different challenges and ensures you don't become overly dependent on any single source of help.

Professional Support Team Members:

Individual Therapist: Mental health professional experienced in personality disorders, trauma recovery, and relationship abuse who can provide ongoing emotional support and skill development.

Psychiatrist: If you're experiencing anxiety, depression, or other mental health symptoms that might benefit from medication, a psychiatrist can provide evaluation and treatment.

Legal Advocate: Attorney or legal advocate who understands domestic violence and family law, available for consultation about legal options and rights.

Financial Advisor: Professional who can help you rebuild financial independence and plan for your future security.

Medical Doctor: Healthcare provider who understands how stress and trauma affect physical health and can address any stress-related health problems.

Personal Support Team Members:

Trusted Friends: People who knew you before your challenging relationship and can provide reality checks and emotional support during difficult times.

Family Members: Relatives who understand your situation and can provide practical and emotional support when needed.

Support Group Members: Other people with similar experiences who can provide understanding and practical advice that friends and family might not be able to offer.

Mentor or Coach: Someone who has successfully navigated similar challenges and can provide guidance and encouragement for your recovery journey.

Spiritual or Religious Leader: If applicable, clergy or spiritual advisors who can provide meaning-making and spiritual support during difficult times.

Building and Maintaining Your Team:

Be Selective: Choose support team members who understand personality disorders or are willing to learn, and who can maintain appropriate boundaries while providing help.

Communicate Your Needs: Help your support team understand what kind of help is most useful and what approaches might be harmful or triggering.

Avoid Over-Reliance: Distribute your support needs among multiple people rather than expecting one person to meet all your emotional or practical needs.

Express Gratitude: Acknowledge the help and support you receive, and look for ways to reciprocate or contribute to others when you're able.

Regular Evaluation: Periodically assess whether your support team is meeting your needs and make adjustments as your situation and recovery progress.

Case Example: Building a Comprehensive Support Network After leaving her relationship with Brian, who had antisocial personality disorder, Lisa realized she needed multiple types of support to rebuild her life safely. Brian had isolated Lisa from many of her friends and family members, so Lisa had to intentionally rebuild her support network from scratch.

Lisa started with professional support, finding a therapist who specialized in narcissistic and antisocial abuse recovery. Lisa also consulted with a legal advocate about restraining orders and financial protection, since Brian had threatened retaliation and had access to Lisa's financial information.

For personal support, Lisa reconnected with her sister and two close friends who had tried to maintain contact despite Brian's interference. Lisa also joined an online support group for survivors of antisocial abuse and eventually participated in a local support group for domestic violence survivors.

Most importantly, Lisa learned to use different support team members for different needs. She used her therapist for processing trauma and developing coping skills, her legal advocate for safety planning and legal questions, her sister for practical help with housing and finances, and her support group for validation and understanding from people with similar experiences.

This diverse support network prevented Lisa from overwhelming any one person with her needs while ensuring she had appropriate help for different aspects of her recovery. Over time, Lisa was able to reduce her reliance on professional support while maintaining the personal relationships that continued to provide meaning and connection in her life.

The Foundation for Your New Life

Recovery from personality disorder relationships isn't a destination— it's an ongoing process of growth, learning, and building the life you want to live. The resources outlined in this chapter provide the framework for that process, but your healing journey will be unique to your circumstances, needs, and goals.

The key to successful recovery lies in using resources strategically rather than trying to access everything at once. Start with the most pressing needs—safety, basic emotional support, and professional guidance—then gradually build additional layers of support as you develop stability and clarity about your direction.

Your investment in appropriate resources and support systems pays dividends not just in your immediate recovery but in your long-term ability to maintain healthy relationships, recognize warning signs, and live with confidence and authenticity. These tools become part of your permanent toolkit for navigating life's challenges with wisdom and strength.

The journey from surviving personality disorder relationships to thriving in healthy connections requires patience, courage, and the right support. With appropriate resources and commitment to your own healing, you can build a life that reflects your values, honors your needs, and provides the security and joy that every person deserves.

Key Resources for Ongoing Success

- Emergency crisis resources provide immediate safety and support during dangerous or overwhelming situations

- Specialized books offer deeper understanding of specific personality disorders and evidence-based coping strategies

- Online communities can provide validation and practical advice when chosen carefully and used with appropriate boundaries

- Technology tools support emotional regulation, pattern tracking, and crisis management through accessible apps and platforms

- Legal resources and advocacy protect your rights and safety when personality disorder relationships involve abuse or high-conflict situations

- Personal support teams provide diverse types of help and prevent over-reliance on any single source of support

Appendix A:All 10 Disorders at a Glance

This comprehensive quick reference provides essential information about each personality disorder, allowing you to quickly identify patterns and understand what you're dealing with in your relationship.

Cluster A: The Odd and Eccentric

Paranoid Personality Disorder

- **Core Pattern**: Pervasive distrust and suspicion of others

- **Key Behaviors**: Surveillance, accusations, hypervigilance about threats

- **Relationship Impact**: Constant questioning of partner's loyalty and motives

- **Partner Experience**: Walking on eggshells, feeling constantly investigated

- **Treatment Outlook**: Poor insight, rarely seeks help voluntarily

- **Red Flags**: Monitoring communications, elaborate conspiracy theories about your activities

- **Boundary Needs**: Consistent limits on surveillance behaviors, documentation of reality

Schizoid Personality Disorder

- **Core Pattern**: Detachment from social relationships and restricted emotional range

- **Key Behaviors**: Emotional unavailability, preference for solitude, limited expression

- **Relationship Impact**: Partner feels like they're dating a ghost

- **Partner Experience**: Loneliness, questioning if they're loved, carrying social burden alone

- **Treatment Outlook**: Limited motivation for change due to comfort with detachment

- **Red Flags**: Complete absence of emotional reciprocity, no interest in shared activities

- **Boundary Needs**: Realistic expectations about emotional availability, maintaining own social life

Schizotypal Personality Disorder

- **Core Pattern**: Eccentric behavior, cognitive distortions, and social anxiety

- **Key Behaviors**: Magical thinking, unusual perceptions, social awkwardness

- **Relationship Impact**: Partner becomes interpreter between them and social world

- **Partner Experience**: Exhaustion from managing social situations, reality confusion

- **Treatment Outlook**: Moderate with therapy focused on social skills and reality testing

- **Red Flags**: Belief in supernatural influences on relationship, social isolation

- **Boundary Needs**: Limits on reality distortion discussions, protection of own social connections

Cluster B: The Dramatic and Emotional

Antisocial Personality Disorder

- **Core Pattern**: Disregard for others' rights, lack of empathy and remorse

- **Key Behaviors**: Manipulation, exploitation, deception, rule-breaking

- **Relationship Impact**: Partner becomes victim of systematic exploitation

- **Partner Experience**: Financial abuse, emotional manipulation, safety concerns

- **Treatment Outlook**: Very poor; lacks motivation for change

- **Red Flags**: Criminal history, financial irregularities, charm followed by exploitation

- **Boundary Needs**: Safety planning, financial protection, often requires leaving

Borderline Personality Disorder

- **Core Pattern**: Instability in relationships, self-image, and emotions

- **Key Behaviors**: Fear of abandonment, emotional dysregulation, impulsivity

- **Relationship Impact**: Intense push-pull dynamics, crisis management

- **Partner Experience**: Emotional exhaustion, walking on eggshells, hypervigilance

- **Treatment Outlook**: Good with DBT and specialized therapy

- **Red Flags**: Threats of self-harm during conflicts, extreme reactions to perceived abandonment

- **Boundary Needs**: Crisis management limits, emotional regulation support

Histrionic Personality Disorder

- **Core Pattern**: Excessive attention-seeking and emotional expression

- **Key Behaviors**: Dramatic displays, constant need for admiration, shallow emotions

- **Relationship Impact**: Partner becomes supporting actor in their performance

- **Partner Experience**: Feeling invisible, exhaustion from constant attention demands

- **Treatment Outlook**: Moderate with therapy focused on emotional regulation

- **Red Flags**: Creating crises for attention, inability to share spotlight

- **Boundary Needs**: Attention-sharing agreements, limits on dramatic behaviors

Narcissistic Personality Disorder

- **Core Pattern**: Grandiosity, need for admiration, lack of empathy

- **Key Behaviors**: Idealization-devaluation cycles, gaslighting, exploitation

- **Relationship Impact**: Partner's reality and self-worth systematically undermined

- **Partner Experience**: Confusion, self-doubt, trauma symptoms

- **Treatment Outlook**: Very poor; lacks insight and motivation

- **Red Flags**: Love-bombing followed by devaluation, gaslighting, entitlement
- **Boundary Needs**: Reality anchoring, often requires leaving for safety

Cluster C: The Anxious and Fearful

Avoidant Personality Disorder

- **Core Pattern**: Social inhibition, feelings of inadequacy, hypersensitivity to rejection
- **Key Behaviors**: Social withdrawal, extreme sensitivity, fear of criticism
- **Relationship Impact**: Partner becomes sole social connection and support system
- **Partner Experience**: Social isolation, responsibility for all external interactions
- **Treatment Outlook**: Good with gradual exposure therapy and support
- **Red Flags**: Complete social avoidance, inability to handle any criticism
- **Boundary Needs**: Gradual independence building, social responsibility sharing

Dependent Personality Disorder

- **Core Pattern**: Excessive need for care and fear of separation
- **Key Behaviors**: Decision-making paralysis, clinging behavior, submission
- **Relationship Impact**: Partner becomes responsible for two lives

- **Partner Experience**: Exhaustion from constant decision-making, loss of autonomy

- **Treatment Outlook**: Good with gradual independence training

- **Red Flags**: Complete inability to function independently, panic during separations

- **Boundary Needs**: Gradual responsibility transfer, decision-making limits

Obsessive-Compulsive Personality Disorder

- **Core Pattern**: Preoccupation with orderliness, perfectionism, and control

- **Key Behaviors**: Rigid standards, workaholic tendencies, inflexibility

- **Relationship Impact**: Partner's efforts never meet impossibly high standards

- **Partner Experience**: Constant criticism, feeling inadequate, loss of spontaneity

- **Treatment Outlook**: Moderate with cognitive therapy focused on flexibility

- **Red Flags**: Impossibly high standards, inability to delegate or relax

- **Boundary Needs**: Standard negotiations, protected time for spontaneity

Appendix B: Emergency Safety Planning Template

Use this template to create a personalized safety plan for crisis situations. Fill out each section and keep copies in multiple secure locations.

Personal Information

- **Your Name:** _____

- **Emergency Contact 1:** _____ (Phone: _____)

- **Emergency Contact 2:** _____ (Phone: _____)

- **Primary Doctor:** _____ (Phone: _____)

- **Therapist/Counselor:** _____ (Phone: _____)

Crisis Resources

- **National Suicide Prevention Lifeline:** 988

- **National Domestic Violence Hotline:** 1-800-799-7233

- **Crisis Text Line:** Text HOME to 741741

- **Local Police:** 911

- **Local Crisis Center:** _____ (Phone: _____)

- **Local Hospital Emergency:** _____ (Phone: _____)

Warning Signs Recognition

When your partner shows these signs, implement safety measures:

- Escalating verbal threats or anger

- Threats of self-harm or suicide

- Property destruction or violence toward objects

- Substance abuse during emotional crisis

- Isolating you from support systems

- Other warning signs specific to your situation:
  _____

Safety Strategies

If you must leave immediately:

1. **Safe location to go**: _____

2. **Transportation plan**: _____

3. **Key you can grab quickly**: _____

4. **Cash location**: _____

5. **Important documents location**: _____

If children are involved:

1. **School emergency contact plan**: _____

2. **Childcare backup**: _____

3. **Child safety conversation plan**: _____

Communication safety:

1. **Safe phone contact**: _____

2. **Code words for help**: _____

3. **Social media safety plan:** _____

Important Documents (Keep copies in safe location)

- Driver's license/ID
- Social Security card
- Birth certificates (yours and children's)
- Passport
- Insurance cards
- Bank account information
- Credit card information
- Lease/mortgage documents
- Medical records
- Medication lists
- Legal documents (restraining orders, custody papers)

Financial Safety

- **Emergency cash location:** _____
- **Safe bank account number:** _____
- **Trusted person who can help financially:** _____
- **Hidden credit card information:** _____

Legal Information

- **Attorney contact:** _____ (Phone: _____)
- **Legal aid organization:** _____ (Phone: _____)

- Restraining order information: _____

- Custody information: _____

After-Crisis Plan

1. Safe place to stay long-term: _____

2. Work notification plan: _____

3. Children's school notification: _____

4. Medical care access: _____

5. Ongoing therapy contact: _____

Review and update this plan every 3 months or after any major changes in your situation.

Appendix C: Communication Scripts for Difficult Conversations

These scripts provide specific language for common challenging situations in personality disorder relationships. Adapt them to your specific circumstances and communication style.

Setting Boundaries Scripts

For Surveillance/Control Behaviors:

- "I understand you feel worried when you don't know where I am. I will check in with you at [specific times], but I won't provide detailed accounts of every interaction I have."

- "I can see that you're feeling anxious about this. I'm not going to discuss this topic anymore tonight. We can talk about it tomorrow when we're both calmer."

- "I've already answered that question, and my answer hasn't changed. I'm not going to keep repeating the same information."

For Emotional Manipulation:

- "I can see you're very upset. I'm not going to make any decisions about our relationship while you're in crisis. Let's talk about this when you're feeling more stable."

- "Your feelings are valid, and threatening to hurt yourself is not an acceptable way to express them. I'm going to call [crisis resource] to make sure you're safe."

- "I understand you're disappointed in my decision. That doesn't change my decision."

For Criticism and Devaluation:

- "I'm not participating in conversations where you're putting me down. When you're ready to discuss this respectfully, I'm happy to talk."

- "I can see you have strong opinions about how I should handle this. This is my decision to make."

- "That comment was hurtful. I need you to speak to me respectfully, or I'll need to take a break from this conversation."

Crisis De-escalation Scripts

For Emotional Meltdowns:

- "I can see you're really struggling right now. I'm here with you, and we're going to get through this."

- "You're safe right now. Let's focus on breathing together. In for four counts, hold for four, out for four."

- "This feeling is temporary, even though it feels overwhelming right now. What's one thing that usually helps you feel a little better?"

For Threats and Ultimatums:

- "I care about you, and I'm not going to make important decisions based on threats. When you're feeling calmer, we can discuss what you need."

- "If you're thinking about hurting yourself, we need to get you professional help right now. That's more important than our relationship discussion."

- "I understand you feel strongly about this. Giving me ultimatums makes it harder for me to consider your concerns."

For Paranoid Accusations:

- "I can see you're feeling scared and suspicious. Those feelings are real, even though I disagree with your interpretation of what's happening."

- "I understand you believe that's true. I have a different understanding of the situation. We seem to see this very differently."

- "I've told you the truth about this situation. I'm not going to keep defending myself against accusations that aren't based in reality."

Ending Conversations Scripts

When Discussion Becomes Circular:

- "We've been discussing this for [time period] and we're not making progress. I need to take a break from this conversation."

- "We seem to be repeating the same points. I'm going to step away for [specific time] and we can try again later if you'd like."

- "I've shared my perspective and heard yours. We disagree, and that's okay. This conversation is over for now."

When You Need Space:

- "I need some time to think about what you've said. I'm going to [specific activity] and we can talk more [specific time]."

- "I'm feeling overwhelmed and need a break. I'll be back in [specific time] and we can continue this if needed."

- "I care about you and I need some space right now. This doesn't mean I'm leaving or that our relationship is over."

Validation Scripts (That Don't Enable)

Acknowledging Feelings Without Agreeing:

- "I can see this situation is really painful for you."

- "It makes sense that you would feel hurt when you interpret things that way."

- "Your emotions are valid, even though I see the situation differently."

- "I understand you're scared. Fear is a normal response when you believe you're in danger."

Supporting Without Rescuing:

- "This sounds like a really difficult decision for you to make. What options are you considering?"

- "I believe in your ability to handle this challenge. What resources do you have available?"

- "That sounds stressful. What do you think would be most helpful for you right now?"

Appendix D: Self-Care Checklist for Overwhelmed Partners

Use this checklist regularly to assess and maintain your emotional, physical, and mental well-being while dealing with personality disorder relationship challenges.

Daily Self-Care Essentials

Physical Care:

- [ ] Got adequate sleep (7-9 hours)
- [ ] Ate regular, nutritious meals
- [ ] Took medications as prescribed
- [ ] Engaged in some form of physical activity
- [ ] Practiced good hygiene and self-care
- [ ] Limited alcohol and avoided drugs
- [ ] Took breaks from screens and technology

Emotional Care:

- [ ] Acknowledged and validated my own feelings
- [ ] Practiced at least one stress-reduction technique
- [ ] Set at least one boundary with my partner
- [ ] Connected with at least one supportive person
- [ ] Engaged in an activity I enjoy
- [ ] Practiced self-compassion rather than self-criticism
- [ ] Avoided isolating myself completely

Mental Care:

- [ ] Challenged any negative self-talk

- [ ] Maintained perspective about my partner's behavior

- [ ] Focused on what I can control vs. what I cannot

- [ ] Made at least one decision based on my own needs

- [ ] Engaged in learning or mental stimulation

- [ ] Practiced mindfulness or present-moment awareness

Weekly Self-Care Assessment

Social Connections:

- [ ] Spent quality time with friends or family

- [ ] Maintained relationships outside my romantic partnership

- [ ] Participated in social activities I enjoy

- [ ] Shared my experiences with someone who understands

- [ ] Avoided isolating myself due to shame or exhaustion

Personal Identity:

- [ ] Engaged in hobbies or interests that are uniquely mine

- [ ] Made progress on personal goals unrelated to my relationship

- [ ] Expressed my authentic self rather than adapting to my partner's needs

- [ ] Maintained my own opinions and preferences

- [ ] Took time for personal reflection and self-discovery

Professional/Life Management:

- [ ] Maintained my work performance and professional relationships

- [ ] Handled personal responsibilities (bills, appointments, etc.)

- [ ] Made progress on long-term goals and plans

- [ ] Maintained my living environment

- [ ] Protected my financial independence

Monthly Self-Care Review

Overall Well-being Assessment:

- [ ] My anxiety levels are manageable most days

- [ ] I feel connected to my authentic self

- [ ] I maintain hope for my future

- [ ] I can identify and express my own needs

- [ ] I have energy for activities beyond managing my relationship

- [ ] I feel supported by others in my life

- [ ] I'm making progress on personal goals

Relationship Impact Assessment:

- [ ] I can distinguish between my partner's emotions and my own

- [ ] I maintain boundaries even when my partner is upset

- [ ] I don't feel responsible for my partner's mental health

- [ ] I can make decisions based on my own values and needs

- [ ] I recognize when my partner's behavior is not my fault

226

- [ ] I have realistic expectations about what I can and cannot change

Red Flag Warning Signs:

- [ ] **Check if experiencing**: Loss of identity or interests

- [ ] **Check if experiencing**: Chronic anxiety or depression

- [ ] **Check if experiencing**: Isolation from friends and family

- [ ] **Check if experiencing**: Financial problems due to relationship

- [ ] **Check if experiencing**: Physical health problems from stress

- [ ] **Check if experiencing**: Inability to make decisions independently

- [ ] **Check if experiencing**: Constant fear of partner's reactions

If you checked multiple red flag items, consider:

- Increasing professional support (therapy, medical care)

- Reconnecting with support systems

- Re-evaluating relationship boundaries

- Consulting with domestic violence resources

- Considering whether the relationship is sustainable

Emergency Self-Care Plan

When Feeling Overwhelmed:

1. **Immediate safety**: Remove yourself from harmful situations

2. **Grounding technique**: Use 5-4-3-2-1 method (5 things you see, 4 you hear, 3 you touch, 2 you smell, 1 you taste)

3. **Breathing**: Practice 4-7-8 breathing (inhale 4, hold 7, exhale 8)

4. **Support contact**: Call someone from your support network

5. **Professional help**: Contact therapist or crisis line if needed

Self-Care Recovery Plan:

- Take at least 24 hours away from relationship stress

- Engage in comforting activities (bath, favorite food, gentle exercise)

- Connect with supportive friends or family

- Practice extra self-compassion

- Consider adjusting boundaries or expectations

- Schedule time with therapist or counselor

Appendix E: Questions to Ask Potential Therapists

Finding the right therapist for personality disorder relationship issues requires asking specific questions to ensure they have appropriate experience and approach. Use these questions during initial consultations.

Experience and Training Questions

General Experience:

- "How many years have you been practicing therapy?"

- "What percentage of your practice involves working with personality disorder relationships?"

- "Have you worked with partners/family members of people with personality disorders, or primarily with the individuals who have the disorders?"

Specific Training:

- "What specific training do you have in personality disorders?"

- "Are you trained in DBT, schema therapy, or other evidence-based approaches for personality disorders?"

- "Do you have experience with the specific personality disorder I'm dealing with?"

- "Have you received training in trauma-informed care?"

Approach and Philosophy:

- "What is your general approach to working with partners of people with personality disorders?"

- "How do you balance supporting the partner while not demonizing the person with the disorder?"

- "Do you believe personality disorders can improve with treatment? What does that process typically look like?"

Practical Approach Questions

Assessment and Planning:

- "How do you typically assess the impact of personality disorder relationships on partners?"

- "What would be your goals for our work together?"

- "How do you help partners distinguish between their own mental health issues and reactions to their partner's behavior?"

- "Do you help with safety planning if needed?"

Specific Interventions:

- "What specific skills or techniques would you teach me for managing relationship stress?"

- "How do you approach boundary-setting in personality disorder relationships?"

- "Do you provide guidance about staying in vs. leaving these relationships?"

- "How do you help partners rebuild their identity and self-esteem?"

Crisis Management:

- "Are you available for crisis situations outside of regular sessions?"

- "How do you handle situations involving threats of self-harm or suicide?"

- "What would you do if you believed I was in physical danger?"

- "Do you coordinate with other professionals (psychiatrists, legal advocates) when needed?"

Red Flag Questions to Assess Therapist Competence

Ask these questions and be concerned if you get the following responses:

Question: "What do you think causes personality disorders?" **Red Flag Answer**: Blaming parents, trauma, or suggesting they're untreatable character flaws **Good Answer**: Multifactorial causes including genetics, brain development, and early experiences; treatable with appropriate intervention

Question: "Should I stay in my relationship or leave?" **Red Flag Answer**: Immediate advice without assessment, or categorical answers like "always leave" or "never give up" **Good Answer**: "That's a decision only you can make. Let's explore what factors are most important to you and help you make an informed choice."

Question: "Is my partner's behavior my fault?" **Red Flag Answer**: Suggesting you caused or contributed to their personality disorder **Good Answer**: Clear explanation that personality disorders develop independently and you're not responsible for causing or curing them

Question: "How do you view people with personality disorders?" **Red Flag Answer**: Stigmatizing language, suggesting they're manipulative or hopeless **Good Answer**: Compassionate but realistic view that acknowledges both suffering and potential for change with treatment

Logistical Questions

Practical Considerations:

- "What are your session fees and what insurance do you accept?"

- "How often would we typically meet?"

- "What is your cancellation policy?"

- "How do you handle communication between sessions?"

- "Do you provide referrals to other professionals if needed (psychiatrists, legal advocates, support groups)?"

Treatment Planning:

- "How long do you typically work with partners dealing with these issues?"

- "How do you measure progress in therapy?"

- "What would indicate that our work together is successful?"

- "At what point would you refer me to someone else or suggest ending therapy?"

Follow-Up Assessment Questions

After 2-3 sessions, evaluate:

- Do you feel understood and supported by this therapist?

- Are you learning practical skills you can use in your daily life?

- Does the therapist maintain appropriate boundaries (not becoming your friend or taking over your decision-making)?

- Do you feel comfortable discussing difficult topics with this therapist?

- Is the therapist helping you maintain perspective rather than either minimizing your experience or encouraging you to see everything as abusive?

Warning signs to consider changing therapists:

- Pushing you toward specific decisions about your relationship

- Seeming overwhelmed or out of their depth with personality disorder issues

- Focusing only on your own behavior without acknowledging your partner's condition

- Providing generic relationship advice that doesn't apply to personality disorder dynamics

- Making you feel worse about yourself or your situation consistently

Appendix F: State-by-State Mental Health Resources

This comprehensive directory provides specific resources for each state, including crisis hotlines, domestic violence services, legal aid, and specialized personality disorder treatment centers.

National Resources (Available in All States)

Crisis Intervention:

- **National Suicide Prevention Lifeline**: 988

- **Crisis Text Line**: Text HOME to 741741

- **National Domestic Violence Hotline**: 1-800-799-7233

- **SAMHSA National Helpline**: 1-800-662-4357

Legal Resources:

- **National Legal Aid & Defender Association**: www.nlada.org

- **Legal Services Corporation**: www.lsc.gov

- **National Coalition Against Domestic Violence**: www.ncadv.org

State-Specific Resources

Alabama

- **Crisis Center**: Alabama Crisis Center Network - 1-800-273-8255

- **Domestic Violence**: Alabama Coalition Against Domestic Violence - (334) 832-4842

- **Legal Aid**: Legal Aid of Alabama - (866) 456-4995

- **Mental Health**: Alabama Department of Mental Health - (334) 242-3454

Alaska

- **Crisis Center**: Careline Alaska - (877) 266-4357

- **Domestic Violence**: Alaska Network on Domestic Violence - (907) 586-3650

- **Legal Aid**: Alaska Legal Services Corporation - (907) 272-9431

- **Mental Health**: Alaska Division of Behavioral Health - (907) 465-3370

Arizona

- **Crisis Center**: Arizona Crisis Line - (602) 222-9444

- **Domestic Violence**: Arizona Coalition to End Sexual & Domestic Violence - (602) 279-2900

- **Legal Aid**: Arizona Legal Aid - (602) 258-3434

- **Mental Health**: Arizona Department of Health Services - (602) 542-1025

Arkansas

- **Crisis Center**: Arkansas Crisis Center - (888) 274-7472

- **Domestic Violence**: Arkansas Coalition Against Domestic Violence - (501) 812-0571

- **Legal Aid**: Arkansas Legal Aid - (501) 376-3423

- **Mental Health**: Arkansas Division of Behavioral Health Services - (501) 686-9164

California

- **Crisis Center**: California Youth Crisis Line - (800) 843-5200

- **Domestic Violence**: California Partnership to End Domestic Violence - (916) 444-7163

- **Legal Aid**: Legal Aid Foundation of Los Angeles - (800) 399-4529

- **Mental Health**: California Department of Health Care Services - (916) 440-7800

- **Specialized**: McLean Hospital West Coast - (855) 856-4773

Colorado

- **Crisis Center**: Colorado Crisis Services - (844) 493-8255

- **Domestic Violence**: Colorado Coalition Against Domestic Violence - (303) 831-9632

- **Legal Aid**: Colorado Legal Services - (303) 837-1313

- **Mental Health**: Colorado Department of Human Services - (303) 866-7400

Connecticut

- **Crisis Center**: Connecticut Crisis Line - (203) 624-3544

- **Domestic Violence**: Connecticut Coalition Against Domestic Violence - (860) 282-7899

- **Legal Aid**: Connecticut Legal Services - (860) 344-0380

- **Mental Health**: Connecticut Department of Mental Health - (860) 418-7000

Delaware

- **Crisis Center**: Delaware Crisis Line - (302) 652-3072

- **Domestic Violence**: Delaware Coalition Against Domestic Violence - (302) 658-2958

- **Legal Aid**: Delaware Legal Aid Society - (302) 575-0660
- **Mental Health**: Delaware Division of Substance Abuse and Mental Health - (302) 255-9399

Florida

- **Crisis Center**: Florida Crisis Line - (833) 456-4566
- **Domestic Violence**: Florida Coalition Against Domestic Violence - (850) 425-2749
- **Legal Aid**: Florida Legal Services - (850) 385-7342
- **Mental Health**: Florida Department of Children and Families - (850) 717-4000

Georgia

- **Crisis Center**: Georgia Crisis & Access Line - (800) 715-4225
- **Domestic Violence**: Georgia Coalition Against Domestic Violence - (404) 209-0280
- **Legal Aid**: Georgia Legal Aid - (833) 457-5399
- **Mental Health**: Georgia Department of Behavioral Health - (404) 657-2252

Hawaii

- **Crisis Center**: Hawaii Crisis Line - (808) 832-3100
- **Domestic Violence**: Hawaii State Coalition Against Domestic Violence - (808) 832-9316
- **Legal Aid**: Legal Aid Society of Hawaii - (808) 536-4302
- **Mental Health**: Hawaii Department of Health - (808) 586-4400

Idaho

- **Crisis Center**: Idaho Crisis Line - (208) 398-4357

- **Domestic Violence**: Idaho Coalition Against Sexual & Domestic Violence - (208) 384-0419

- **Legal Aid**: Idaho Legal Aid Services - (208) 746-7541

- **Mental Health**: Idaho Department of Health and Welfare - (208) 334-5500

Illinois

- **Crisis Center**: Illinois Crisis Line - (217) 359-4141

- **Domestic Violence**: Illinois Coalition Against Domestic Violence - (217) 789-2830

- **Legal Aid**: Legal Aid Chicago - (312) 341-1070

- **Mental Health**: Illinois Department of Human Services - (217) 557-1601

Indiana

- **Crisis Center**: Indiana Crisis Line - (800) 273-8255

- **Domestic Violence**: Indiana Coalition Against Domestic Violence - (317) 917-3685

- **Legal Aid**: Indiana Legal Services - (317) 631-9410

- **Mental Health**: Indiana Division of Mental Health - (317) 232-7800

Iowa

- **Crisis Center**: Iowa Crisis Line - (855) 581-8111

- **Domestic Violence**: Iowa Coalition Against Domestic Violence - (515) 244-8028

- **Legal Aid**: Iowa Legal Aid - (800) 532-1275

- **Mental Health**: Iowa Department of Human Services - (515) 281-5032

Kansas

- **Crisis Center**: Kansas Crisis Line - (888) 363-2287

- **Domestic Violence**: Kansas Coalition Against Sexual and Domestic Violence - (785) 232-9784

- **Legal Aid**: Kansas Legal Services - (785) 233-2068

- **Mental Health**: Kansas Department for Aging and Disability Services - (785) 296-4986

Kentucky

- **Crisis Center**: Kentucky Crisis Line - (800) 273-8255

- **Domestic Violence**: Kentucky Coalition Against Domestic Violence - (502) 209-5382

- **Legal Aid**: Kentucky Legal Aid - (502) 584-1254

- **Mental Health**: Kentucky Cabinet for Health and Family Services - (502) 564-4527

Louisiana

- **Crisis Center**: Louisiana Crisis Line - (800) 273-8255

- **Domestic Violence**: Louisiana Coalition Against Domestic Violence - (225) 752-1296

- **Legal Aid**: Southeast Louisiana Legal Services - (504) 529-1000

- **Mental Health**: Louisiana Department of Health - (225) 342-9500

Maine

- **Crisis Center**: Maine Crisis Line - (888) 568-1112

- **Domestic Violence**: Maine Coalition to End Domestic Violence - (207) 941-1194

- **Legal Aid**: Maine Legal Services for the Elderly - (207) 622-4731

- **Mental Health**: Maine Department of Health and Human Services - (207) 287-3707

Maryland

- **Crisis Center**: Maryland Crisis Line - (410) 531-6677

- **Domestic Violence**: Maryland Network Against Domestic Violence - (301) 352-4574

- **Legal Aid**: Maryland Legal Aid - (410) 951-7777

- **Mental Health**: Maryland Department of Health - (410) 767-6860

Massachusetts

- **Crisis Center**: Massachusetts Crisis Line - (877) 382-1609

- **Domestic Violence**: Jane Doe Inc. - (617) 248-0922

- **Legal Aid**: Massachusetts Legal Assistance Corporation - (617) 367-8544

- **Mental Health**: Massachusetts Department of Mental Health - (617) 626-8000

- **Specialized**: McLean Hospital (Original) - (617) 855-2000

Michigan

- **Crisis Center**: Michigan Crisis Line - (800) 273-8255

- **Domestic Violence**: Michigan Coalition to End Domestic Violence - (517) 347-7000

- **Legal Aid**: Michigan Legal Services - (517) 487-5148
- **Mental Health**: Michigan Department of Health and Human Services - (517) 373-3740

Minnesota

- **Crisis Center**: Minnesota Crisis Line - (800) 273-8255
- **Domestic Violence**: Minnesota Coalition for Battered Women - (651) 646-6177
- **Legal Aid**: Minnesota Legal Aid - (651) 842-7301
- **Mental Health**: Minnesota Department of Human Services - (651) 431-2000

Mississippi

- **Crisis Center**: Mississippi Crisis Line - (877) 210-8513
- **Domestic Violence**: Mississippi Coalition Against Domestic Violence - (601) 981-9196
- **Legal Aid**: Mississippi Center for Legal Services - (601) 948-6752
- **Mental Health**: Mississippi Department of Mental Health - (601) 359-1288

Missouri

- **Crisis Center**: Missouri Crisis Line - (800) 273-8255
- **Domestic Violence**: Missouri Coalition Against Domestic Violence - (573) 634-4161
- **Legal Aid**: Legal Services of Eastern Missouri - (314) 534-4200
- **Mental Health**: Missouri Department of Mental Health - (573) 751-4122

Montana

- **Crisis Center**: Montana Crisis Line - (877) 688-3377

- **Domestic Violence**: Montana Coalition Against Domestic Violence - (406) 443-7794

- **Legal Aid**: Montana Legal Services Association - (406) 442-9830

- **Mental Health**: Montana Department of Public Health - (406) 444-3622

Nebraska

- **Crisis Center**: Nebraska Crisis Line - (800) 273-8255

- **Domestic Violence**: Nebraska Coalition to End Sexual and Domestic Violence - (402) 476-6256

- **Legal Aid**: Nebraska Legal Aid - (402) 348-1069

- **Mental Health**: Nebraska Department of Health and Human Services - (402) 471-3121

Nevada

- **Crisis Center**: Nevada Crisis Line - (775) 784-8090

- **Domestic Violence**: Nevada Coalition to End Domestic Violence - (775) 828-1115

- **Legal Aid**: Nevada Legal Services - (702) 386-1070

- **Mental Health**: Nevada Division of Public and Behavioral Health - (775) 684-4200

New Hampshire

- **Crisis Center**: New Hampshire Crisis Line - (603) 668-6111

- **Domestic Violence**: New Hampshire Coalition Against Domestic Violence - (603) 224-8893

- **Legal Aid**: New Hampshire Legal Assistance - (603) 224-3333

- **Mental Health**: New Hampshire Department of Health and Human Services - (603) 271-5000

New Jersey

- **Crisis Center**: New Jersey Crisis Line - (855) 654-6735

- **Domestic Violence**: New Jersey Coalition for Battered Women - (609) 584-8107

- **Legal Aid**: Legal Services of New Jersey - (732) 572-9100

- **Mental Health**: New Jersey Division of Mental Health Services - (609) 777-0702

New Mexico

- **Crisis Center**: New Mexico Crisis Line - (855) 662-7474

- **Domestic Violence**: New Mexico Coalition Against Domestic Violence - (505) 246-9240

- **Legal Aid**: New Mexico Legal Aid - (505) 266-5680

- **Mental Health**: New Mexico Behavioral Health Services - (505) 476-9266

New York

- **Crisis Center**: New York State Crisis Line - (800) 273-8255

- **Domestic Violence**: New York State Coalition Against Domestic Violence - (518) 482-5465

- **Legal Aid**: Legal Aid Society - (212) 577-3300

- **Mental Health**: New York State Office of Mental Health - (518) 474-4403

North Carolina

- **Crisis Center**: North Carolina Crisis Line - (800) 273-8255

- **Domestic Violence**: North Carolina Coalition Against Domestic Violence - (919) 956-9124

- **Legal Aid**: Legal Aid of North Carolina - (866) 219-5262

- **Mental Health**: North Carolina Department of Health and Human Services - (919) 855-4800

North Dakota

- **Crisis Center**: North Dakota Crisis Line - (800) 273-8255

- **Domestic Violence**: North Dakota Council on Abused Women's Services - (701) 255-6240

- **Legal Aid**: Legal Services of North Dakota - (701) 746-8405

- **Mental Health**: North Dakota Department of Human Services - (701) 328-8920

Ohio

- **Crisis Center**: Ohio Crisis Line - (877) 275-6364

- **Domestic Violence**: Ohio Domestic Violence Network - (614) 781-9651

- **Legal Aid**: Ohio Legal Services - (614) 241-2001

- **Mental Health**: Ohio Department of Mental Health - (614) 466-2596

Oklahoma

- **Crisis Center**: Oklahoma Crisis Line - (800) 273-8255

- **Domestic Violence**: Oklahoma Coalition Against Domestic Violence - (405) 557-1210

- **Legal Aid**: Legal Aid Services of Oklahoma - (918) 584-3211

- **Mental Health**: Oklahoma Department of Mental Health - (405) 522-3908

Oregon

- **Crisis Center**: Oregon Crisis Line - (800) 273-8255

- **Domestic Violence**: Oregon Coalition Against Domestic Violence - (503) 365-9644

- **Legal Aid**: Oregon Legal Aid - (503) 302-9708

- **Mental Health**: Oregon Health Authority - (503) 945-5944

Pennsylvania

- **Crisis Center**: Pennsylvania Crisis Line - (855) 284-2494

- **Domestic Violence**: Pennsylvania Coalition Against Domestic Violence - (717) 545-6400

- **Legal Aid**: Pennsylvania Legal Aid Network - (717) 236-9486

- **Mental Health**: Pennsylvania Department of Human Services - (717) 787-6443

Rhode Island

- **Crisis Center**: Rhode Island Crisis Line - (401) 414-4357

- **Domestic Violence**: Rhode Island Coalition Against Domestic Violence - (401) 467-9940

- **Legal Aid**: Rhode Island Legal Services - (401) 274-2652

- **Mental Health**: Rhode Island Department of Behavioral Healthcare - (401) 462-2339

South Carolina

- **Crisis Center**: South Carolina Crisis Line - (833) 364-2274

- **Domestic Violence**: South Carolina Coalition Against Domestic Violence - (803) 256-2900

- **Legal Aid**: South Carolina Legal Services - (803) 744-9430

- **Mental Health**: South Carolina Department of Mental Health - (803) 898-8581

South Dakota

- **Crisis Center**: South Dakota Crisis Line - (800) 273-8255

- **Domestic Violence**: South Dakota Coalition Ending Domestic Violence - (605) 945-0869

- **Legal Aid**: East River Legal Services - (605) 336-9230

- **Mental Health**: South Dakota Department of Social Services - (605) 773-5990

Tennessee

- **Crisis Center**: Tennessee Crisis Line - (855) 274-7471

- **Domestic Violence**: Tennessee Coalition to End Domestic Violence - (615) 386-9406

- **Legal Aid**: Legal Aid Society of Middle Tennessee - (615) 244-6610

- **Mental Health**: Tennessee Department of Mental Health - (615) 532-6500

Texas

- **Crisis Center**: Texas Crisis Line - (832) 416-1177

- **Domestic Violence**: Texas Council on Family Violence - (512) 794-1133

- **Legal Aid**: Texas Legal Services Center - (512) 477-6000

- **Mental Health**: Texas Health and Human Services - (512) 424-6500

Utah

- **Crisis Center**: Utah Crisis Line - (801) 587-3000

- **Domestic Violence**: Utah Domestic Violence Coalition - (801) 521-5544

- **Legal Aid**: Utah Legal Services - (801) 328-8891

- **Mental Health**: Utah Department of Human Services - (801) 538-4270

Vermont

- **Crisis Center**: Vermont Crisis Line - (802) 229-0001

- **Domestic Violence**: Vermont Network Against Domestic Violence - (802) 223-1302

- **Legal Aid**: Vermont Legal Aid - (802) 863-5620

- **Mental Health**: Vermont Department of Mental Health - (802) 651-1557

Virginia

- **Crisis Center**: Virginia Crisis Line - (855) 635-0595

- **Domestic Violence**: Virginia Sexual & Domestic Violence Action Alliance - (804) 377-0335

- **Legal Aid**: Virginia Legal Aid Society - (866) 534-5243

- **Mental Health**: Virginia Department of Behavioral Health - (804) 786-3921

Washington

- **Crisis Center**: Washington Crisis Line - (866) 427-4747

- **Domestic Violence**: Washington State Coalition Against Domestic Violence - (206) 389-2515

- **Legal Aid**: Northwest Justice Project - (888) 201-1014

- **Mental Health**: Washington State Department of Health - (360) 236-4200

West Virginia

- **Crisis Center**: West Virginia Crisis Line - (304) 623-4357

- **Domestic Violence**: West Virginia Coalition Against Domestic Violence - (304) 965-3552

- **Legal Aid**: West Virginia Legal Services - (304) 342-6814

- **Mental Health**: West Virginia Department of Health - (304) 558-0627

Wisconsin

- **Crisis Center**: Wisconsin Crisis Line - (608) 280-2600

- **Domestic Violence**: Wisconsin Coalition Against Domestic Violence - (608) 255-0539

- **Legal Aid**: Wisconsin Legal Services - (608) 256-3304

- **Mental Health**: Wisconsin Department of Health Services - (608) 266-9622

Wyoming

- **Crisis Center**: Wyoming Crisis Line - (888) 279-7790

- **Domestic Violence**: Wyoming Coalition Against Domestic Violence - (307) 755-5481

- **Legal Aid**: Wyoming Legal Services - (307) 632-3699

- **Mental Health**: Wyoming Department of Health - (307) 777-7094

Specialized Treatment Centers by Region

Northeast:

- McLean Hospital (Massachusetts) - (617) 855-2000

- New York Presbyterian (New York) - (212) 305-6001

- Sheppard Pratt (Maryland) - (410) 938-3000

Southeast:

- Menninger Clinic (Texas) - (713) 275-5000

- Pine Rest (Michigan) - (616) 455-9200

- Skyland Trail (Georgia) - (404) 851-5438

Midwest:

- Laureate Psychiatric Clinic (Oklahoma) - (918) 481-4000

- Timberline Knolls (Illinois) - (630) 293-3540

- Rogers Behavioral Health (Wisconsin) - (800) 767-4411

West:

- Avalon Hills (Utah) - (855) 417-8266

- Monte Nido (California) - (888) 228-1253

- Cognitive Behavioral Institute (California) - (858) 357-4325

This comprehensive resource guide provides the foundation for accessing appropriate help regardless of your location or specific needs. Keep these resources easily accessible and don't hesitate to reach out when you need support—seeking help is a sign of strength, not weakness.

References

1. Agrawal, H.R., Gunderson, J., Holmes, B.M. and Lyons-Ruth, K., 2004. Attachment studies with borderline patients: A review. *Harvard Review of Psychiatry*, 12(2), pp.94-104.

2. Bateman, A. and Fonagy, P., 2019. Handbook of mentalizing in mental health practice. *American Journal of Psychiatry*, 176(4), pp.272-281.

3. Bender, D.S., Dolan, R.T., Skodol, A.E., Sanislow, C.A., Dyck, I.R., McGlashan, T.H., Shea, M.T., Zanarini, M.C., Oldham, J.M. and Gunderson, J.G., 2001. Treatment utilization by patients with personality disorders. *American Journal of Psychiatry*, 158(2), pp.295-302.

4. Biskin, R.S. and Paris, J., 2012. Management of borderline personality disorder. *Canadian Medical Association Journal*, 184(17), pp.1897-1902.

5. Bornovalova, M.A., Hicks, B.M., Iacono, W.G. and McGue, M., 2009. Stability, change, and heritability of borderline personality disorder traits from adolescence to adulthood: A longitudinal twin study. *Development and Psychopathology*, 21(4), pp.1335-1353.

6. Clarkin, J.F., Yeomans, F.E. and Kernberg, O.F., 2006. Psychotherapy for borderline personality disorder: Focusing on object relations. *Journal of Clinical Psychology*, 62(4), pp.445-461.

7. Crawford, T.N., Cohen, P., First, M.B., Skodol, A.E., Johnson, J.G. and Kasen, S., 2008. Comorbid Axis I and Axis II disorders in early adolescence: Outcomes 20 years later. *Archives of General Psychiatry*, 65(6), pp.641-648.

8. Crowell, S.E., Beauchaine, T.P. and Linehan, M.M., 2009. A biosocial developmental model of borderline personality: Elaborating and extending Linehan's theory. *Psychological Bulletin*, 135(3), pp.495-510.

9. Feenstra, D.J., Bushman, B.J., Kersten, T., Luman, M. and Koenigs, M., 2011. Angry words on angry faces: Enhanced attention to emotional faces in borderline personality disorder. *Clinical Psychological Science*, 1(4), pp.414-428.

10. Fonagy, P., Gergely, G., Jurist, E. and Target, M., 2018. Affect regulation, mentalization and the development of the self. *Journal of the American Psychoanalytic Association*, 66(2), pp.289-318.

11. Grant, B.F., Chou, S.P., Goldstein, R.B., Huang, B., Stinson, F.S., Saha, T.D., Smith, S.M., Dawson, D.A., Pulay, A.J., Pickering, R.P. and Ruan, W.J., 2008. Prevalence, correlates, disability, and comorbidity of DSM-IV borderline personality disorder. *Journal of Clinical Psychiatry*, 69(4), pp.533-545.

12. Gunderson, J.G. and Lyons-Ruth, K., 2008. BPD's interpersonal hypersensitivity phenotype: A gene-environment-developmental model. *Journal of Personality Disorders*, 22(1), pp.22-41.

13. Haslam, N., Holland, E. and Kuppens, P., 2012. Categories versus dimensions in personality and psychopathology: A quantitative review of taxometric research. *Psychological Medicine*, 42(5), pp.903-920.

14. Hoffman, P.D., Fruzzetti, A.E. and Buteau, E., 2007. Understanding and engaging families: An education, skills and support program for relatives impacted by borderline personality disorder. *Journal of Mental Health*, 16(1), pp.69-82.

15. Johnson, J.G., Cohen, P., Brown, J., Smailes, E.M. and Bernstein, D.P., 1999. Childhood maltreatment increases risk for personality disorders during early adulthood. *Archives of General Psychiatry*, 56(7), pp.600-606.

16. Kernberg, O.F., 2012. The inseparable nature of love and aggression: Clinical and theoretical perspectives. *International Journal of Psychoanalysis*, 93(4), pp.851-870.

17. Lenzenweger, M.F., Lane, M.C., Loranger, A.W. and Kessler, R.C., 2007. DSM-IV personality disorders in the National Comorbidity Survey Replication. *Biological Psychiatry*, 62(6), pp.553-564.

18. Linehan, M.M., Comtois, K.A., Murray, A.M., Brown, M.Z., Gallop, R.J., Heard, H.L., Korslund, K.E., Tutek, D.A., Reynolds, S.K. and Lindenboim, N., 2006. Two-year randomized controlled trial and follow-up of dialectical behavior therapy vs therapy by experts for suicidal behaviors and borderline personality disorder. *Archives of General Psychiatry*, 63(7), pp.757-766.

19. Links, P.S., Heslegrave, R. and van Reekum, R., 1999. Impulsivity: Core aspect of borderline personality disorder. *Journal of Personality Disorders*, 13(1), pp.1-9.

20. Lyons-Ruth, K., Yellin, C., Melnick, S. and Atwood, G., 2005. Expanding the concept of unresolved mental states: Hostile/helpless states of mind on the Adult Attachment Interview are associated with disrupted mother-infant communication and infant disorganization. *Development and Psychopathology*, 17(1), pp.1-23.

21. McMain, S.F., Links, P.S., Gnam, W.H., Guimond, T., Cardish, R.J., Korman, L. and Streiner, D.L., 2009. A randomized trial of dialectical behavior therapy versus general psychiatric

management for borderline personality disorder. *American Journal of Psychiatry*, 166(12), pp.1365-1374.

22. Oldham, J.M., 2006. Borderline personality disorder and suicidality. *American Journal of Psychiatry*, 163(1), pp.20-26.

23. Paris, J., 2008. Treatment of borderline personality disorder: A guide to evidence-based practice. *Journal of Psychiatric Practice*, 14(4), pp.243-250.

24. Rosenthal, M.Z., Gratz, K.L., Kosson, D.S., Cheavens, J.S., Lejuez, C.W. and Lynch, T.R., 2008. Borderline personality disorder and emotional responding: A review of the research literature. *Clinical Psychology Review*, 28(1), pp.75-91.

25. Skodol, A.E., Gunderson, J.G., McGlashan, T.H., Dyck, I.R., Stout, R.L., Bender, D.S., Grilo, C.M., Shea, M.T., Zanarini, M.C., Morey, L.C. and Sanislow, C.A., 2002. Functional impairment in patients with schizotypal, borderline, avoidant, or obsessive-compulsive personality disorder. *American Journal of Psychiatry*, 159(2), pp.276-283.

26. Trull, T.J., Jahng, S., Tomko, R.L., Wood, P.K. and Sher, K.J., 2010. Revised NESARC personality disorder diagnoses: Gender, prevalence, and comorbidity with substance dependence disorders. *Journal of Personality Disorders*, 24(4), pp.412-426.

27. Widiger, T.A. and Trull, T.J., 2007. Plate tectonics in the classification of personality disorder: Shifting to a dimensional model. *American Psychologist*, 62(2), pp.71-83.

28. Young, J.E., Klosko, J.S. and Weishaar, M.E., 2003. Schema therapy: A practitioner's guide. *Journal of Cognitive Psychotherapy*, 17(4), pp.365-384.

29. Zanarini, M.C., Frankenburg, F.R., Reich, D.B. and Fitzmaurice, G., 2012. Attainment and stability of sustained symptomatic remission and recovery among patients with borderline personality disorder and axis-II comparison subjects: A 16-year prospective follow-up study. *American Journal of Psychiatry*, 169(5), pp.476-483.

30. Zimmerman, M., Rothschild, L. and Chelminski, I., 2005. The prevalence of DSM-IV personality disorders in psychiatric outpatients. *American Journal of Psychiatry*, 162(10), pp.1911-1918.

www.ingramcontent.com/pod-product-compliance
Lightning Source LLC
Chambersburg PA
CBHW061006280326
41935CB00009B/856